THE
ANTI-AGING
HORMONES

Also by the Author

Super Soy

A Consumer's Guide to Medicines in Food

A Consumer's Dictionary of Medicines

A Consumer's Dictionary of Cosmetics Ingredients

A Consumer's Dictionary of Food Additives

A Consumer's Dictionary
of Household, Yard, and Office Chemicals

Poisons in Your Food

Ageless Aging

Cancer-Causing Agents

How to Reduce Your Medical Bills

THE
ANTI-AGING
HORMONES

THAT CAN HELP YOU BEAT THE CLOCK

BENEFITS AND DANGERS OF
MELATONIN • HUMAN GROWTH HORMONE
DHEA • ESTROGEN • TESTOSTERONE
INSULIN • LEPTIN • THYROID
GROWTH FACTORS

RUTH WINTER, M.S.

THREE RIVERS PRESS
NEW YORK

Endocrine illustration on page 15 and second illustration on page 10 courtesy of LifeART Collection Images, copyright © 1989–1996 by TechPool Studios, Cleveland, Ohio. Illustration on page 6 and first illustration on page 10 by Jennifer Harper.

Published by Three Rivers Press, a division of Crown Publishers, Inc., 201 East 50th Street, New York, New York 10022. Member of the Crown Publishing Group.

Random House, Inc. New York, Toronto, London, Sydney, Auckland
http://www.randomhouse.com/

Three Rivers Press and colophon are trademarks of Crown Publishers, Inc.

Printed in the United States of America

Design by Mercedes Everett

Library of Congress Cataloging-in-Publication Data

Winter, Ruth, 1930–
    The anti-aging hormones that can help you beat the clock :
  benefits and dangers of : melatonin, human growth hormone, DHEA,
  estrogen, testosterone, insulin, leptin, thyroid, growth factors /
  Ruth Winter, — 1st ed.
       p.   cm.
    Includes bibliographical references and index.
    1. Longevity.   2. Aging—Hormone therapy.   I. Title.
  RA776.75.W54 1997
  612.6′7—dc21   97-12228
                                                         CIP

ISBN 0-609-80015-9

10 9 8 7 6 5 4 3 2 1

First Edition

To Arthur Winter, M.D., my personal physician

CONTENTS

ACKNOWLEDGMENTS

The author wishes to thank Samuel Dower, M.D., associate director of the Joslin Clinic and endocrinologist on the staff of St. Barnabas Medical Center, Livingston, New Jersey, and all the other busy researchers who gave of their valuable time to describe for this book their exciting investigations.

THE
ANTI-AGING
HORMONES

HORMONES
TO BEAT THE CLOCK

How old are you?

How fast are you aging?

Your answers lie not in the date your mother gave birth to you nor with the number of wrinkles on your face. Your true age is ordained by extremely potent chemicals your body manufactures, known as hormones.

Tremendous research efforts are now under way, fueled by the federal government, pharmaceutical manufacturers, and universities, to identify, understand, and use hormones to prevent or reverse signs we associate with aging. The stakes are high because the largest generation in U.S. history and one-third of our present population—the "baby boomers"—will begin turning sixty-five years old in 2011.[1]

Ultimately, however, the boomers will find themselves part of another major demographic movement—the explosive growth in the numbers of very old people living to age eighty-five and beyond. From 1960 to 1994, these "oldest old," who in large portion are quite frail and poor, have increased by 274 percent. Their numbers are expected to reach nearly 7 million by 2020 and soar to at least 19 million and possibly to 27 million or higher by 2050.[2]

Phyllis Moen, Ph.D., the Ferris Family Professor of Life

Course Studies at Cornell University and codirector of the Cornell Applied Gerontology Research Institute, points out that Americans can now expect to spend up to one-third of their lives beyond retirement and that by the year 2030 there will be more Americans over age sixty-five than children under eighteen. "Yet, our research indicates that about half of retirees retire unexpectedly with little or no planning and that the retirement transition is extraordinarily diverse, not at all a routinized exit." She calls the stage "limbo," because it describes their predicament so well.[3]

The number of old people is not as important as their health and vitality. If they can be youthful, active, and productive, it will benefit not only them but the younger generation, who could then avoid the financial and emotional burdens of caring for millions of sick, dependent elderly, including their parents, grandparents, and even great-grandparents.

Can we beat the clock and stay youthful, happy, and healthy?

Hormones are our body's timekeepers. They are major principals in determining how long and how well we will live.

What are hormones? The word *hormone* is derived from the Greek word *hormao,* meaning "I arouse to activity." Hormones are secreted by our endocrine glands, which spurt them directly into our bloodstream. Although a hormone may be circulated throughout our body, it affects only a specific target organ or organs. It is not unlike a direct telephone call. The more of the hormone in our blood usually the more active the target organ becomes. The amount of the hormone released depends upon our body's needs. If the feedback from our body is faulty or the endocrine glands fail to produce enough of the needed hormone upon demand, all sorts of physical and mental disorders may occur. This hormonal imbalance happens to all of us as we age but in some faster than in others.

The largest of the hormone secretors, the pancreas, has an

average weight of less than three ounces. The smallest, the mysterious pineal, is about the size of a grape seed. All the others together—the thyroid, the four parathyroids, the twin adrenals, the pituitary, the thymus, and the paired ovaries of women or testes of men—weigh between four and seven ounces. Yet, as tiny as they are, these mighty glands oversee our lives and behavior. They control the digestion of our food and its transformation into blood, bone, muscles, and brain. They make us tall or short, fat or thin. They regulate our heartbeat and affect the workings of our liver and kidneys. They set the time when a girl becomes a woman and a boy a man. They determine fertility, sexual behavior, and personality. When we are attacked by a foe—either human or germ—they mobilize our defenses.

All the hormone secretors work in concert. They are a grand chemical orchestra that when playing harmoniously keeps us healthy and happy. But as time goes by, some of the players weaken and become discordant, and we develop signs we associate with aging—such as weakened immunity, wrinkled skin, ebbing muscular strength, insomnia, and loss of sexual desire.

New understanding of how hormones—some long identified and others newly discovered—perform is leading to great strides in beating the clock. Scientists are now able—better than ever before—to measure hormone levels as we age. Researchers are gaining more and more understanding of what causes the deterioration of the body as we live year by year, and they are attempting to prevent or reverse some of the changes by replacing what is lost with natural or synthetic hormones. The catch is, however, that because these chemicals are so powerful in minute amounts and work in such exquisite balance, supplementing one or two may throw off the harmony of the rest, sometimes resulting in disasters such as cancers or heart attacks. Furthermore, hormones are not the only factors in aging. While they may time "biological clocks" and affect all our organs and tissues, heredity, wear and tear, and exposure to environmental conditions all play roles in how long and how well we live.

This book is an effort to provide you with information about the latest advances in endocrine research. Scientists today are so rapidly identifying hormones within the body and then creating hormone products that new information was being received all the time I was writing this manuscript. Many of the terms and the concepts will be new to you. Even if you were recently graduated from high school or college, or even graduate school, much of the material in this book is too recently developed for you to have encountered it during your formal education. If you don't understand or forget the meaning of a term as you go through the book, you don't have to rush out and take a hormone. Hopefully, I remembered to put it in the glossary.

As you will read, chances are excellent that modern versions of the long-sought "fountain of youth" are bubbling in a number of the nation's top research laboratories.

1. THE CHEMICALS THAT CONTROL YOUR RIPENING

They Are Literally in Your Head

There's an old army saying: "If it's the bugler's job to wake up the camp each morning, whose job is it to wake up the bugler?"

The pituitary was considered the bugler—the master gland that sent out the messages to endocrine glands all over your body such as your sex glands and your thyroid to wake them up and to put them to sleep. Then, in the 1960s it was discovered that the one who woke up the bugler was a portion of your brain known as the *hypothalamus*. This tiny cluster of cells provides a link between the "thinking" part of your brain *(cerebral cortex)* and your pea-sized pituitary gland in the center of your skull behind the bridge of your nose.

There is no greater proof that your mind and your body cannot be separated than the fully integrated feedback system involving your hypothalamus, your pituitary, and all your other endocrine glands. This system responds to and affects everything that happens within and without your body. It reacts to what you perceive as pleasure or danger. It affects how healthy you are and how much you enjoy your life. And it is this system that many believe controls your aging and your lifespan.

While this chapter may contain some complicated words and explanations, it is vital you make the effort to understand

MAJOR HORMONE PRODUCERS

The chemicals that control body rhythms, functions and aging. Several other organs also manufacture hormones: the stomach, the liver, intestines, kidneys, and heart all contain groups of hormone-secreting cells.

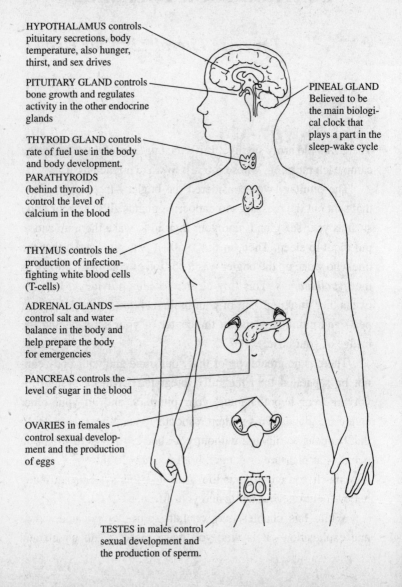

HYPOTHALAMUS controls pituitary secretions, body temperature, also hunger, thirst, and sex drives

PITUITARY GLAND controls bone growth and regulates activity in the other endocrine glands

THYROID GLAND controls rate of fuel use in the body and body development.
PARATHYROIDS (behind thyroid) control the level of calcium in the blood

THYMUS controls the production of infection-fighting white blood cells (T-cells)

ADRENAL GLANDS control salt and water balance in the body and help prepare the body for emergencies

PANCREAS controls the level of sugar in the blood

OVARIES in females control sexual development and the production of eggs

PINEAL GLAND
Believed to be the main biological clock that plays a part in the sleep-wake cycle

TESTES in males control sexual development and the production of sperm.

the exciting new scientific discoveries about what is happening in your body. Your well-being and even your life may depend upon it.

Your nervous system and your hormonal system do interact with each other and share control of your body. They both secrete chemical messengers and send them to target organs and tissues in your body. They differ, however, in two ways:

First, your hormones act slowly and their effects are long lasting, whereas your nervous system acts quickly and produces almost instantaneous responses.

Second, your hormonal system pours its products directly into your bloodstream, while your nervous system uses sequences of nerves to communicate directly with target organs and tissues.

Your hypothalamus—this intermediary between your brain and your body—plays a role in the way you move and in your emotions and motivations. Sleep, pleasure, eating, reproductive behavior, and stress-related aggression all emanate from this tiny area. It is a message center for your senses. When you see a person who is sexually attractive to you or you experience a painful cut or smell freshly baked bread, your hypothalamus becomes aware of it and so do you. This message center also possesses information about things outside your awareness, such as the level of hormones in your blood and the concentration of nutrients in your body.

Your hypothalamus replies to state-of-the-body messages partly through your pituitary gland, which then sends out its chemical orders that turn on and turn off your other endocrine glands. There is an amazing and exquisite feedback between the one who "wakes up the bugler," your hypothalamus, and the "bugler," your pituitary, which are connected by a stalk, and the rest of your endocrine glands. When you experience emotional disturbances such as anxiety and worry, you can interfere with this communication and cause an imbalance in your hormones and thus a disturbance in your body. Physical disorders within the hypothalamus, on the other hand, may produce conditions such as sexual precocity, lack of appetite, enormous obesity, or premature aging.

Virtually all hormones produced by the hypothalamus and the pituitary are emitted in a burstlike fashion with brief periods of inactivity and activity interspersed in a definite circadian rhythm—about a twenty-four-hour schedule—with increased secretion during specific hours of the day. Certain hormones involved in the menstrual cycle, however, have a more frequent rhythm.

Didn't you ever wonder why you were more alert and energetic at one period of the day than another or one time of the month than another or even one season of the year? It's your hormonal clocks at work.

Your hypothalamus secretes various *releasing* and *inhibiting* hormones that order your pituitary to send out or hold back its own "turn on" and "turn off" chemical signals to target organs. Thus far, six hypothalamic chemical "commands" to the pituitary have been identified:

Thyrotropin-releasing hormone (TRH) stimulates your pituitary to release a hormone that chemically "pokes" your thyroid gland into releasing its hormone. TRH was reported in 1996 to have shown effectiveness in helping to combat nerve damage in animals, and in a small clinical study of patients with spinal cord injury, its effectiveness was reported as promising.[1]

Gonadotropin-releasing hormone (GnRH), also known as luteinizing hormone–releasing hormone (LH-RH), orders your pituitary to spew hormones that target your sex glands, and they then emit their own hormones.

Dopamine inhibits a number of your pituitary's hormones. Dopamine is also a nerve messenger (a neurotransmitter), and it serves as a basic material from which you make your own stimulants. When something interferes with the production of dopamine, movements may become involuntary, such as the shaking of the head and hands of patients with Parkinson's disease, a chronic, progressive, degenerative disorder of the central nervous system that does not usually occur until after the age of forty-five.

Corticotropin-releasing hormone (CRH) stimulates the release of ACTH, which affects your adrenal glands.

Growth hormone–releasing hormone (GHRH) encourages your pituitary to release growth hormone. GHRH is one of the hottest substances being studied as an anti-aging hormone!

Somatostatin *inhibits* the release of both growth hormone and thyroid-stimulating hormone from your pituitary. In the pancreas, somatostatin can also *inhibit* insulin secretion.

Chances are your brain's hypothalamus contains other powerful chemical substances not yet identified, as does your pituitary, sitting in its protected "Turk's saddle" (sella turcica) in your head behind your nose.

Your pituitary has two storage places for hormones awaiting orders from your hypothalamus: the back portion, the *posterior pituitary,* and the front portion, the *anterior pituitary.* There is a *middle* portion. In animals, it secretes melanocyte-stimulating hormone (MSH), which temporarily darkens the skin of cold-blooded creatures for camouflage. The center pituitary is also involved in aggressive and mating behavior in animals. Its purpose in humans has not yet been identified.

The following are the known powerful executive hormones from your pituitary and what their recognized jobs are.

In the anterior pituitary:

ACTH (adrenocorticotropic hormone) stimulates the release of hormones from your adrenal glands above your kidneys including cortisol (produced as a medicine in 1952 to treat severe inflammation). The interaction of your hypothalamus, your pituitary, and your adrenal gland plays a large part in your stress reactions (see chapter 2).

Gonadotropins target the testes and ovaries. The follicle-stimulating hormone (FSH) *stimulates* the development of the ovaries and the production of sperm cells as well as brings about the maturation of an egg cell in its little follicle or capsule on the ovary. Luteinizing hormone in females stimulates the ovary and brings about the incredible journey of the egg down the tubes to the womb. In males it stimulates the secretion of testosterone by the testes.

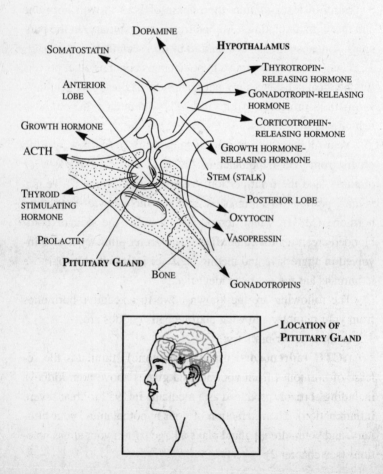

Prolactin stimulates the breasts to produce milk.

Thyroid-stimulating hormone causes your thyroid gland to release its hormones.

Growth hormone (somatotropin), as its name implies, regulates physical growth and metabolism. As you will read in chapter 3, this may be one of the most important "anti-aging" hormones.

In the posterior pituitary:

Oxytocin, vital in childbirth and nursing, targets the breast and the smooth muscles of the uterus.

Vasopressin (antidiuretic hormone) promotes water conservation by the kidneys. At high concentrations, it also causes the blood vessels to constrict, and it is being studied for its effects on memory and learning. The reason beer and whiskey increase the frequency of urination is that alcohol slows the secretion of vasopressin, whose job it is to help your body conserve water. Lack of vasopressin or the kidneys' inability to react to it also results in diabetes insipidus. In this condition, a person is extremely thirsty and takes in and excretes extreme amounts of water.

When the pituitary gland overproduces growth hormone, there is excessive growth in all parts of the body. If it underproduces hormones from the front portion of the gland, the result is sexual underdevelopment or infertility, premature aging, a generalized weakness, and often general ill health.

Your endocrine glands affect your mood and brain function. If you are a woman—or you have lived with a woman—who has suffered from premenstrual tension or postpartum depression, you know how dramatically hormones can affect mood. Men with high levels of male hormones—naturally or by supplementation—can be very aggressive.

Your hypothalamus, your pituitary, and your other endocrine glands turned you from a baby into an adult. They help you digest and use your food and do other important things, not the least of which is keeping you alive. Measurements of hormone levels through the stages of life show that all decline, some more than others. But as the Scottish writer George Macdonald so aptly put it at the turn of the last century, "Age is not all decay; it is the ripening, the swelling, of the fresh life within, that withers and bursts the husks."

Summing it up, a number of hypothalamic, pituitary, and sex hormones have been identified and then manufactured in the laboratory. They are used in therapy for a variety of human ills. They are now being studied as a means of not only treating but preventing many of the conditions we associate with aging, as you will read in the following chapters. As more is learned about these extremely powerful "executive chemicals" in our bodies, we will be able to ripen with much less decay.

2. STRESS AND MAINTAINING YOUTHFUL IMMUNITY

DHEA and Thymus Hormones

Why does our immunity break down as the years go by?

Dr. Hans Selye, the famed director of the University of Montreal's Institute of Experimental Medicine, had an explanation.

"A motor car doesn't suddenly cease running because of old age. It stops because of failure of some part that has worn out. It is the same with people. Under continuous stress—either physical or mental—some vital body part gives way, leading to a variety of illnesses, and eventually death."[1]

Dr. Selye's stress theory is one of the twentieth century's major medical milestones. He found the body's endocrine glands—particularly the adrenals—strive to maintain equilibrium within the body. When any threat occurs either inside or outside the body, the glands react instantly. The adrenals release "stress" hormones such as epinephrine (formerly called adrenaline). The stress hormones cause the blood pressure and blood sugar to rise, stomach acid to increase, and the arteries to tighten. We are then prepared to fight or flee.

As the danger—real or imagined—abates, "calming" hormones take over, such as cortisone from the adrenals and ACTH from the pituitary. This was the "resistance" phase, according to

Dr. Selye. But if the hormonal tug-of-war occurs too often, we become exhausted and vulnerable to all sorts of ills.

Since Dr. Selye's defining of the "stress response," scientists have learned more and more about the hormonal interaction we humans undergo when we are threatened.

Our two adrenal glands sit right above our kidneys. Each adrenal is about one to two inches long and weighs just a fraction of an ounce. Each is also divided into two parts. One is the outer layer, the *cortex*. When you are stressed, your hypothalamus in your brain secretes CRH (corticotropin-releasing hormone). CRH causes your pituitary gland in your head to secrete a burst of ACTH (adrenocorticotropin hormone). ACTH, in turn, stimulates the outside of your adrenal gland to emit glucocorticoid hormones into your bloodstream to raise your blood sugar and give you added energy. Those substances emitted by your adrenal's outer layer, such as the glucocorticoid hormones, are called *steroids*. There are three principal types:

1. *Mineralocorticoids,* whose job it is to control the balance of sodium and potassium in the body.
2. *Glucocorticoids,* that monitor the level of sugar in the blood.
3. *Sex hormones.*

The second part of your adrenal is the middle, the *medulla*. It responds to the nervous system and what you perceive to be alarming. This inner portion of your adrenal secretes two hormones, epinephrine (adrenaline) and norepinephrine (noradrenaline). They spurt out when you are afraid or angry, to make your heart beat faster and let your lungs take in more air.

One of the major hormones from the outer portion of your adrenal gland is *cortisol,* also known as *hydrocortisone*. Stress may cause your adrenals to secrete twenty times the usual amount of cortisol, and this prepares you to deal with trouble by mobilizing "defenses." It wrenches amino acids out of your muscles and other tissues, helps send them to your liver, and there it speeds their conversion into an emergency supply of blood sugar. It also releases fatty acids from your fat tissues. How all this helps in your stress reaction is not entirely known, but it is clear that your adrenal hormones prepare you for fight or flight.[2]

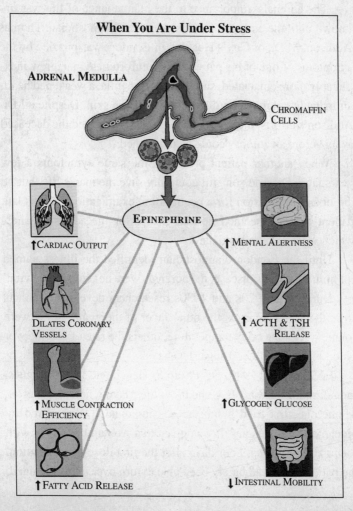

When You Are Under Stress

ADRENAL MEDULLA

CHROMAFFIN CELLS

EPINEPHRINE

↑CARDIAC OUTPUT

↑ MENTAL ALERTNESS

DILATES CORONARY VESSELS

↑ ACTH & TSH RELEASE

↑MUSCLE CONTRACTION EFFICIENCY

↑GLYCOGEN GLUCOSE

↑ FATTY ACID RELEASE

↓ INTESTINAL MOBILITY

ARE YOU UNDERGOING ADRENOPAUSE?

Does this powerful alarm system eventually overstress your organs and literally wear you out, or is there another phenomenon—*adrenopause?* In the latter—just as in menopause—the adrenal glands, like the ovaries, stop producing a youthful amount of their hormones, and the result is certain signs we associate with aging, such as loss of strength and heart trouble.

The adrenals' importance to the maintenance of life was unknown until the early 1850s, when a super diagnostician, Thomas Addison, M.D., of Guy's Hospital in London, was puzzled by the symptoms of one of his patients. The unfortunate man grew inexplicably more emaciated, suffered from anemia, a weakened heart, an irritable colon, and a discoloration of the skin. Despite all Dr. Addison's efforts, the man died. The family whisked the deceased away before an autopsy could be performed.[3]

When another patient presented the same symptoms a few years later, Dr. Addison still could not save the man's life, but he did obtain permission for a postmortem examination. All his late patient's organs seemed normal except for the adrenal glands, which were withered and hard.

Until the London diagnostician identified the illness named for him, Addison's disease, the adrenals were not considered vital.

During the 1920s and 1930s researchers developed extracts from the adrenal cortex, the outer layer of the gland. Some were found to regulate body temperature, others the rate of heartbeat or blood pressure or blood sugar levels.

In September 1948, Dr. Philip S. Hench and his colleagues, including Dr. Edward E. Kendall, at the Mayo Clinic, Rochester, Minnesota, first tried a substance, compound E, discovered by biochemist Dr. Kendall. It was given to a woman bedridden with rheumatoid arthritis. Four days after the first dose of medication, the patient, who had barely been able to turn over in bed unaided, dressed herself and, to everyone's utter amazement, went downtown on a three-hour shopping spree.

Her physicians, Merck & Co.—the pharmaceutical firm that had prepared the medication—the press, and in fact the world were excited. An adrenal hormone had been found that could alleviate symptoms of rheumatoid arthritis. In less than two months, compound E—now known as cortisone—had severe effects in the dosage used initially. While cortisone and its relatives are in wide use today to relieve inflammation and swelling, physicians now know that it can have serious consequences such as weakening the immune system, making bones fragile, and causing other physical and emotional problems if not used in small doses over a short time.[4]

More than forty-six hormones are now known to be secreted by the adrenals. Many of our current medicines for inflammatory and autoimmune diseases are real or factory-made imitations of adrenal products. John F. Kennedy, as a young senator from Massachusetts, suffered from Addison's disease and would certainly never have captured the Presidency if it hadn't been for the availability of supplemental adrenal hormones to combat his life-threatening symptoms.

DHEA—Aging Controller?

In addition to the stress hormones that may play a part in aging us, another more recently discovered adrenal hormone, DHEA (dehydroepiandrosterone), is causing a stir at this writing with some media proclaiming it the long-sought "fountain of youth."

Dr. Etienne-Emile Baulieu, developer of the controversial RU-486 "abortion pill," created a sensation in Paris in 1995 when a cover story in the French weekly *Le Point* described his work with an "anti-aging pill" containing DHEA.[5] Baulieu, somewhat startled by the worldwide interest, stressed that the pill would not extend life but might, after further testing, enable people to "age well."

Many researchers are enthusiastic about DHEA therapy because the body converts it to a variety of hormones that decline with age, including those governing sexual and immune functions.

DHEA production peaks during the midtwenties. By around age thirty, levels begin to taper off until, by eighty, most people have less than one-fifth the DHEA they had in their youth. Why would the body produce such an abundance of a hormone—it is the most plentiful steroid hormone in the human body—then suddenly tighten the tap? No one knows. But researchers suspect the decline may be part of the reason we show signs of aging.[6]

That some people lose less DHEA than others may explain why some seem to age better than others. At any time in life, DHEA levels can differ dramatically from person to person. It tends to be lower among adults with diabetes, high blood pressure, Alzheimer's, heart disease, impotence, bladder cancer, lupus, multiple sclerosis, and other disorders.[7]

Do low levels of DHEA help cause these problems? If so, will taking it help reverse or prevent them?

DHEA THERAPY

In laboratory animals, DHEA seems to protect against a number of cancers—breast, liver, lung, colon, skin, prostate, testicular, and ovarian. When pregnant rats received whole-body irradiation and were implanted with DES (diethylstilbestrol, a female hormone) 96.2 percent developed breast cancer. But when the pregnant rats were given DHEA and irradiated, the incidence of breast tumors decreased by 35 percent and the malignancies that did occur did so five months later than those in the untreated rats.[8]

DHEA also reportedly sharpens memory in animals, keeps atherosclerosis and autoimmune diseases from turning severe, and strengthens virus defenses. In animals the hormone also seems to act like an "anti-aging pill." Mice prone to obesity stay slim and lean—and live longer—when given doses of 500 mg per kilogram of body weight of DHEA three times a week. DHEA did not suppress their appetite, indicating it speeded up their metabolism. The decrease in body fat was primarily due to a decrease in the number of fat cells. DHEA reportedly did not cause any toxic effects.[9]

A certain strain of mouse develops diabetes. When the strain was given 0.4 percent DHEA in their diet, their diabetes was rapidly reversed. Other experimental animals have shown similar results.[10]

When older mice were put on a regular DHEA regimen, their cells were found to attack infectious agents as well as did the cells from young mice. Old mice on DHEA even looked young: their thick, shiny coats and energy made them hard to distinguish from animals half their age.[11]

Will it do the same for us humans?

Since France's Dr. Baulieu first encountered DHEA more than three decades ago, only a few small studies of DHEA in humans have been completed, although many are under way.

In a study published in the *New England Journal of Medicine* in 1986, Dr. Samuel Yen, a leading DHEA researcher, an endocrinologist, and his colleagues at Medical School of the University of California at San Diego measured DHEA levels in 242 men fifty to seventy-nine years old, then tracked their health for twelve years. Men whose initial levels were higher than 140 mcg per deciliter of blood were less than half as likely to have died of heart disease by the end of the study, even when researchers took into account such factors as smoking and cholesterol levels. Those with the highest levels fared the best. For every hundred-point increase, there was a 48 percent drop in heart disease risk and a 36 percent decrease in death by any cause.[12]

France's Dr. Baulieu reported similar findings.[13] He tested fifty-seven subjects and found DHEA is a "good individual marker of age." As people age, he says, "everybody's level diminishes. But somebody who has a lot of DHEA to start with will maintain a fairly high count, while those who had a low level in the beginning will always be in the lowest category."

Dr. Yen and his group reported in 1995 that giving thirty elderly people small doses of DHEA daily for six months improved their well-being, which Dr. Yen defines as "the ability to cope." Less than 10 percent reported feeling better while on a placebo. Among the other results of the DHEA therapy were increased mobility, less joint discomfort, sounder sleep, a boost in immune function, and a decrease in fat.[14]

"This is not a fountain of youth. It is not going to make you live longer," said Dr. Yen, trying to temper the mounting excitement after announcing his results at the first conference on DHEA and aging, held in Washington, D.C., in 1995. "It is a drug that may help people age gracefully."[15]

Dr. Yen is currently giving DHEA to another group of older patients to determine whether it will halt or reverse the natural decline in their strength and muscle mass.

Dr. Baulieu plans, as of this writing, to analyze blood samples from six hundred elderly people, trying to correlate DHEA levels and general health. And he hopes soon to begin testing small doses of the hormone on as many as two hundred volunteers, measuring any changes in memory, behavior, skin and muscle tone, cholesterol levels, cardiac activity, and joint pain.

Dr. William Regelson, coauthor of the best-seller *The Melatonin Miracle* with Walter Pierpaoli, M.D., Ph.D. (New York: Pocket Books, 1995), is also enthusiastic about DHEA. In an article in the *Sciences,* September 1995, Dr. Regelson is quoted as saying, "In 1982, my mother-in-law had a midthigh amputation and became markedly weak, depressed, senile as a post. Here she was, living in my house, essentially a vegetable. So I threw everything at her except the kitchen sink. It wasn't a study; it was an act of desperation. But lo and behold, when I gave her DHEA, she became a normal human being again."[16]

Dr. Regelson's wife also has reportedly been taking DHEA ever since, and he started taking it more than five years ago.

He and his colleagues at the Medical College of Virginia theorize that DHEA may act by buffering or antagonizing the action of corticosteroids to modify stress-mediated injury to tissue.[17] This is the action that Dr. Selye also maintained may be critical to the degenerative disease of aging.

In a study of healthy subjects from sixty-four to over eighty-five and young controls, twenty to forty, Dr. Regelson and his colleagues found an "intriguing inverse relationship" between DHEA and cardiovascular mortality in men, as Dr. Yen had found. In women from the same population, however, the Virginia researchers found that mortality from heart disease in women was highest among those with the highest DHEA levels.[18]

Drs. Regelson and Kalimi say in the preface of their textbook, *Biologic Role of Dehydroepiandrosterone (DHEA)*, published by Walter deGrutyer & Co. in 1990, that for many years the study of DHEA focused on its role as an intermediate in sex-steroid production. More recently, they report, DHEA or related analogs, have been found to prevent cancer and to show action against diabetes. They note there is growing interest in DHEA therapy for hardening of the arteries, high blood pressure, failing memory, disorders of fat mobilization, and cancer prevention and treatment. One of its most important abilities is, they claim, that DHEA may bolster immunity to viral or bacterial infections. It may also act in ways similar to the heart stimulant digitalis. As if that weren't enough, the doctors say that it may be useful in fatigue syndromes and in lowering blood cholesterol.[19]

Dr. Regelson admits many uncertainties concerning the role

of DHEA in the nervous, immune, and endocrine networks have yet to be unraveled, and the question remains whether the age-related decrease of DHEA is related to the failure of specific organs such as the adrenals or the sex glands or whether it results from changes in feedback or regulatory mechanisms. DHEA is one of the few compounds that shows a gradual decrease with advancing age, reaching an asymptomatic low at the age of maximum recorded life span.

"This raises the possibility of DHEA being one of the cogwheels of the hypothetical clock which determines life span," Dr. Regelson says.

The University of Virginia investigator notes variation in response to DHEA in immune studies depends on the dose and route of administration, which suggests that DHEA is processed by the body into several active substances including the sex hormones estrogen and androgen.

Clinical trials—that means DHEA is actually being given to patients under strict medical guidelines—are under way for treatment of cancer, obesity, high cholesterol, Alzheimer's, and multiple sclerosis.

DHEA is now being tested to revitalize the ailing immune systems of the elderly. At the University of Utah Medical Center in Salt Lake City, Raymond Daynes, Ph.D., clinical professor and associate director of research at the Geriatric Research Education and Clinical Center at the Veterans Administration Medical Center, Salt Lake City, believes that DHEA can make vaccinations more effective in older people.[20]

He has proven that hepatitis vaccine is more effective in old rats when their DHEA is brought up to youthful levels. At the University of Rochester, Dr. Thomas Evans, associate clinical professor of medicine, tested whether DHEA could shore up the response of elderly persons to flu vaccine. He said the results were promising in a preliminary trial, but that there would have to be more subjects in a DHEA–flu vaccine study before a firm conclusion could be made.[21]

Dr. Daynes has an explanation of why supplemental DHEA could work to shore up immunity in the elderly:

"In the 1990s, we began a series in our laboratory to determine some of the alterations that take place in the immune system of elderly individuals. What we discovered was not a deficiency, but rather the change was mediated through abnormal overproduction of certain molecules. What we found was happening in the average person is that their immune system was slowing down and reaction to a threat was at a much slower pace.

"Some cytokines [substances released by certain cells upon contact with an 'enemy' that act as go-betweens in the immune response] cause inflammation. These cytokines, we found, were being overproduced in an abnormal fashion.

"One of these cytokines, we found, was *IL-6* [*interleukin-6*], which can be protective when produced normally but when overproduced may destroy bone and/or can cause clotting and consequently lead to arthritis, osteoporosis, heart attacks, and strokes. In elderly mice, we found it can also target elderly bone marrow cells and cause lymphomas [a type of immune-system cancer such as the one that killed Jackie Onassis]. When cytokines go out of whack, elderly people can also become overwhelmed by new infectious invaders."

He cautioned that cytokines—those immunity players—have a cascade effect and there is much to learn about them.

What causes the cytokines to go out of whack and what can be done about it?

Dr. Daynes and his colleagues believe it is those old devils *free radicals*. These are molecules that are "single" and looking for partners. It's not unlike the singles ads placed in publications. Sometimes a person who answers an ad is dangerous. The most common and potentially hazardous free radicals are oxygen singles that look for a mate by stealing someone else's partner or by attaching themselves to a couple. Just like the "other" woman or man, they cause a lot of disturbances and destroy relationships. They can deform and corrode any partner they touch. A large body of evidence suggests free radicals can directly and indirectly cause substantial damage to cells lining blood vessels and arteries.[22] Platelets (small, colorless disks circulating in blood that play a part in clotting) tend to gather at the site of injury. This leads to deposits of fibrin, a protein in the blood that enmeshes blood cells to form clots. Cholesterol also gets stopped at the site—all of which contributes to the plugging of blood vessels.

Free radicals have their good side. They play a big part in our ability to kill microbes, and without them we would be helpless to break down food, twitch a muscle, think a thought, or reach for vitamins. Free radicals are controlled with extraordinary precision by our bodies, and usually they are kept in line. It is only when we age or under conditions of abnormal stress that reactive radicals escape the bounds of disciplined performance and begin nicking our cells to pieces.

Dr. Daynes says when he and his colleagues administer DHEA and vitamin E—both potent *antioxidants*—to old rodents, their immune systems return to more youthful levels. DHEA and vitamin E are effective against the oxygen radicals.

Dr. Daynes believes those individuals whose levels of DHEA-sulfate are below one hundred micrograms per hundred deciliters of blood—and this can be tested at most laboratories—are not making enough. He said that some individuals have normal levels even at sixty and seventy years.

He says other researchers have found that DHEA can also inhibit the release of glucocorticoids, the stress hormones generated by the adrenal gland.

How much supplemental DHEA would be beneficial in humans?

Dr. Daynes says, "I personally believe those individuals with DHEA below one hundred micrograms per deciliter of blood could take from twenty-five to fifty milligrams per day forever and it wouldn't hurt them. However, when you get up to one to four grams—which is what some people are taking—then there is the potential for problems with long-term use. Such doses potentially can damage the liver and even cause liver cancer."

Following are other human ills for which DHEA is under study.

AIDS. Researchers at the National Institute of Mental Health and the Division of Biology, California Institute of Technology in Pasadena, found the length of survival after the onset of initial AIDS symptoms is consistent with the normal blood levels of DHEA, in that survival of older people and young children is less than that of young adults. The researchers point out that DHEA reaches its maximum level in young adulthood, and the level of the DHEA in seventy-year-olds is about 20 percent of that found in young adults.[23] Other researchers have found that DHEA is lower in AIDS patients and that it has some potentially therapeutic benefits. In one study done at Temple University, DHEA was found to inhibit AZT-resistant strains of the AIDS virus.[24]

DHEA was given to AIDS patients at California Pacific Medical Center, San Francisco. The compound was well tolerated, and there was some decrease in blood neopterin, a substance from the immune system that is present in high levels as a result of a viral infection, particularly AIDS.[25] The researchers concluded that more studies with DHEA should be done. Since aging impairs immunity, older people may also benefit from results from AIDS studies with DHEA.

Systemic Lupus Erythematosus. Physicians in California are testing DHEA as a possible therapy for systemic lupus erythematosus, a chronic inflammatory disease that primarily strikes young women. Lupus is the classic example where side effects of treatment can be as bad as the disease. Sometimes lupus can only be controlled with massive doses of steroids and anticancer chemotherapy agents. Steroid side effects include weakening of the bones (osteoporosis), an increased risk for diabetes, and other problems that often occur in middle age and beyond. Lupus, like rheumatoid arthritis, is an autoimmune disease. If DHEA can produce results more gently for lupus victims than conventional steroid medication, it may also prove to be beneficial for chronic inflammatory problems that occur during aging.

James McGuire, M.D., chief of staff at Stanford University Hospital and Dr. van Vollenhoven, M.D., professor of rheumatology at Stanford, tested DHEA in fifty-seven women with lupus. The participants took 50 to 200 mg of oral DHEA every day for three to twelve months. About two-thirds reported some relief of symptoms including rashes, joint pain, headaches, and fatigue. Most women in the study said both their ability to concentrate and their tolerance for exercise improved.[26] The Japanese are also testing DHEA in patients with lupus because they believe low blood levels of DHEA may cause deficient production of IL-2 (interleukin-2), a natural substance that transmits signals between types of white blood cells.[27]

Arthritis. Rheumatoid arthritis is an autoimmune disease, that is, a disease in which environmental and/or genetic factors trigger an uncontrollable and destructive reaction by the immune system, directed against the body's own tissue. Population studies have indicated that approximately 1 percent of the adult population is affected with rheumatoid arthritis. The female-to-male ratio is about two to one, and the peak age of incidence is thirty-five to fifty-five in males and forty to sixty in females.[28]

DHEA levels have been found to be low in women with rheumatoid arthritis, a condition frequently associated with osteoporosis. In a study of forty-nine postmenopausal women with rheumatoid arthritis, DHEA levels were significantly lower than in healthy controls. DHEA levels were reduced to an even greater extent in women taking corticosteroids for their arthritis than in those who were not. Usually, corticosteroid medications are synthetic adrenal hormones, such as prednisone and dexamethasone, to treat inflammation. The finding that they reduce DHEA levels is not surprising, since administering corticosteroids is known to reduce the levels of adrenal hormones, as pointed out above. However, DHEA levels were also significantly reduced in arthritic women who were not receiving corticosteroids, but corticosteroid therapy appears to make DHEA deficiency worse.[29]

Studies like this suggest that DHEA might be of benefit to people with rheumatoid arthritis. Corticosteroids are known to be an important cause of osteoporosis; indeed, that is one of the main reasons doctors are so reluctant to prescribe these drugs. Perhaps one of the reasons corticosteroids cause osteoporosis is that they deplete DHEA.

Would simultaneous administration of DHEA inhibit some of the side effects of corticosteroids, including osteoporosis?

Our natural adrenal secretions contain both of these hormones, and nature usually does things for a reason. Animal studies suggest that DHEA does in fact modulate some of the effects of corticosteroids. It appears then that supplementation with DHEA might, indeed, prevent the osteoporosis that so often develops in individuals with rheumatoid arthritis, particularly in those who are taking corticosteroids.

Osteoporosis. Hungarian researchers studied 105 women between the ages of forty-five and sixty-nine and found a definite correlation between DHEA and aging bones. Dr. S. Miklos and colleagues at the Department of Medicine, Semmelweis University, Budapest, found blood levels of DHEA were significantly lower in women with osteoporosis than in those with normal bones. The serum level of DHEA decreased significantly with age in both groups, the Hungarian investigators said. They also found that DHEA did not seem to affect the level of estrogen in the women's bodies and that it may be a useful indicator of low bone mineral density in peri- and postmenopausal women.[30]

Not all prominent researchers believe DHEA is a factor in osteoporosis and aging. Dr. E. Barrett-Connor and her colleagues at the department of Community and Family Medicine, University of California at San Diego, for example, measured the DHEA-sulfate levels in the bones of 260 men and 162 women who were residents of Rancho Bernardo, California. DHEA-S levels had previously been measured in 1972–74 when the men were fifty to seventy years old and the women were fifty-five to seventy-four. In 1988–91, the participants' bone mineral density was again measured. Among the men, DHEA levels and bone mineral density at the hip and in the leg significantly decreased with increasing age. However, for both men and women, there was no significant association of DHEA levels with bone mineral density at any site both before and after adjustment for age, obesity, cigarette smoking, and use of high blood pressure medication. These data do not support the hypothesis that DHEA has a causal role in osteoporosis of the aging, Dr. Barrett-Connor says.[31]

The role of DHEA in fragile bones in aging still remains to be defined. As mentioned above, DHEA can be converted by the body into other hormones. Of particular interest to researchers is DHEA's conversion into estrogen and testosterone, both hormones known to play a role in prevention of bone loss.

Chronic Fatigue Syndrome. This debilitating condition was first described in the 1980s. Its cause is still unknown, although a viral infection is the most suspected culprit. During the past several years, a number of doctors have begun giving DHEA to individuals whose levels are low normal or below normal. In some cases, anecdotal reports say there is improvement in energy levels and general well-being. Since chronic fatigue may also occur during aging, results of studies with DHEA and chronic fatigue syndrome may be of benefit.

Cancer. In contrast to estrogen, which may promote cancer under certain circumstances, DHEA shows promise as an anticancer agent. In a strain of mice that develops spontaneous breast cancer, long-term administration of DHEA prevented the cancer from occurring. Still other investigators indicate an association between DHEA levels and human breast cancer. In one study, urinary excretion of DHEA was below normal in a group of premenopausal women with breast cancer. Other researchers confirmed that DHEA levels are low in premenopausal breast cancer patients but found that some postmenopausal women with breast cancer had elevated DHEA levels. It appeared that the low levels in the premenopausal patients were due primarily to decreased production, while the elevated levels in the postmenopausal patients were due to delayed breakdown. Whatever the reason for the changes, these studies suggest a possible role for DHEA in the prevention or treatment of at least some cases of breast cancer.[32]

Dr. William Regelson and his colleagues Dr. Mohammed Kalimi and Roger Loria, from the Medical College of Virginia, believe DHEA is a "sensitive indicator that can distinguish normal women from patients at risk with breast cancer."[33]

As for colon cancer, treatment of mice with DHEA also

delayed the appearance of colon tumors resulting from administration of a powerful cancer-causing agent (1-2-dimethylhydrazine). In addition, administering DHEA inhibited the development of liver cancer in rats treated with chemical carcinogens.

The question of whether DHEA prevents or plays a part in cancer is still not clear. The adrenal hormone seems to have an anticancer effect by blocking certain enzymes, the workhorses of the cells that change substances into other forms.

Drs. Regelson, Kalimi, and Loria say that subnormal blood and urinary-excretion levels of DHEA have been reported to indicate high risk for breast cancer and evidence of poor prognosis. However, they say, breast cancer patients with high DHEA/cortisol blood ratios respond well to endocrine therapy. They point out that DHEA found in the breast fluid of normal premenopausal and postmenopausal women exceeds that of blood plasma by fifty to a thousand times. It has been suggested, because of this, that high local levels of DHEA can lead to estrogen production in the body that promotes tumor growth. In ovarian tumors, the circulating levels of DHEA are clinically lower than normal, with the lowest values found in ovarian cancer.[34]

Although largely superseded clinically by the use of estrogen blockers, sex steroids have a long history in suppressing the growth of breast tumors. In support of this, DHEA can modulate certain human breast cancer cell growth, which it inhibits by estrogen-metabolizing enzymes. The Virginia researchers said that in their long-term treatment of patients, two renal cancers appeared to have an arrest of progressive disease, one for two and a half years, but no tumor regression was seen.

DHEA has also been reported to have a protective effect on mice when given up to sixteen hours before radiation, and the protective effect lasted for thirty days. In contrast, if given twenty to fifty-two hours before radiation, DHEA showed a radiation-sensitizing action.[35]

A Piece of the Psoriasis Puzzle. Psoriasis is a chronic disease of the skin of unknown cause, usually persisting for years with periods of remission and recurrence. It is characterized by elevation lesions in various parts of the body that are covered with dry, silvery scales that drop off. DHEA has been found to be decreased in the skin of psoriatics. This has led to a wide range of successful topical studies of DHEA in skin detergent preparations with evidence of up to 50 percent absorption in twenty-four hours. DHEA has also been shown to have some success in preventing the appearance of psoriatic lesions when skin inflammation or injury occur in susceptible individuals.[36]

Hair Loss and DHEA. DHEA has been associated with hairiness or hair loss in women. A correlation has also been found between DHEA levels and male-pattern baldness in young men. And, researchers have reported that hair contains high quantities of DHEA.[37] Whether these observations will lead to a new anti-hair-loss product remains to be seen.

Weight Loss and DHEA. Does DHEA increase longevity in animals because it reduces weight? Arthur Schwartz, Ph.D., professor of microbiology at the Fells Institute for Cancer Research at Temple University, says DHEA suppresses the development of many cancers and age-related diseases, just as long-term underfeeding does.

However, the steroid hormone, Dr. Schwartz says, seems to directly prevent some diseases and not just because it effects weight loss.

The DHEA–weight loss–longevity connection is still not clear, and studies are continuing to find answers.[38]

What about Adverse Effects?

In this world, everything comes with a price. Is the cost of DHEA's anti-aging benefits too high?

DHEA is a steroid hormone and a building material for testosterone and estrogen, and excess amounts of these hormones from DHEA may be linked to increased risk for growth of breast and prostate cancers. A study at Oregon State University published in the December 1995 issue of the *Journal of Carcinogenesis* indicated that DHEA triggered tumors in rainbow trout. The trout were given half the clinical daily dose given to humans. In lab animals fed large doses, liver cancer has occurred, but the doses are far greater than the comparable amounts contemplated for humans.

Little is actually known about DHEA's role in the body. One unknown is the body's ability to convert DHEA into different forms, each of which may have varying effects. A second concern is that the bulk of DHEA in the body is in the form of DHEA-sulfate, which may function differently from the unsulfated form of the hormone. Unanswered questions include whether DHEA and its sulfate simply serve as storage pools for the manufacture of estrogen and testosterone, or whether these substances also have biological properties of their own. Because of these uncertainties, scientists don't know whether DHEA is directly responsible for many of the beneficial effects claimed for it, or if the beneficial effects result from DHEA's conversion to estrogen and testosterone.

There are concerns, but so far no adverse effects of moderate doses, meaning 20 to 100 mg a day, have been reported.

San Diego's Dr. Yen saw no adverse effects in his study. People with kidney cancer or multiple sclerosis who have taken extremely high doses—6 to 8 g per day—have not been reported to have had major problems.

Frank Bellino, Ph.D., Endocrinology Program administrator of the National Institute on Aging, says that Dr. Yen's work has been interesting, but one of the problems is Dr. Yen hasn't tried other androgens and estrogens that the body can make from DHEA.

"We don't know whether it's an androgen or estrogen giving the results," Dr. Bellino says, "and reports of 'feeling better' raise the possibility of bias. Some of the biologic parameters don't change much, and it is hard to know if Dr. Yen is measuring the right compound. There seems to be a gender difference, and DHEA effects seem to be more pronounced in men. The muscle strength of women was stronger on the placebo."

Dr. Bellino says his program at NIA has given three grants to study DHEA.

"The grantees are looking at why DHEA declines with age. They are not looking at what happens when you supplement it."

He noted that a pharmaceutical firm is testing DHEA for the treatment of Alzheimer's.

Dr. Bellino acknowledges the work in animals with DHEA is tantalizing. In the rodents, it has reversed Type II diabetes, the kind that usually appears in overweight, middle-aged humans. DHEA has also been shown in rodents to inhibit lung, breast, and skin cancers, promote weight loss by increasing metabolism and suppressing appetite, improve memory, and decrease stress.

Dr. Bellino says, "There is a strong potential for side effects. There are indications that it might cause liver problems. DHEA is a precursor for estrogen and testosterone, and excess amounts of these hormones derived from DHEA may be linked to increased risk for breast and prostate cancers. High testosterone levels in women can lead to excessive facial-hair growth and changes in blood fats, which increase the risk for heart disease.

"So far, DHEA hasn't shown such side effects. But because

the body uses the hormone to make testosterone and estrogen, the side effects and risks of those hormones may hold for DHEA as well. Testosterone in high doses, for example, can cause . . . oily skin and acne in women."

DHEA is available in health food stores, the University of Utah's Dr. Daynes points out: "If you wish to buy such a product over the counter, make sure it says 'DHEA' and not 'a precursor of DHEA.' The latter is not effective at all."

Schiff, a division of Weider Nutrition Group of Salt Lake City, Utah, put pharmaceutical-grade tablets of DHEA on the market in August 1996 in thirty- and sixty-count bottles at the suggested retail price of $6.99 and $12.99 respectively.

No one knows how many people are taking the hormone, but doctors at a DHEA conference at the New York Academy of Sciences in the early 1990s put the number in the thousands.[39] As word of mouth grows, business is bound to get brisker. Just compare DHEA to human growth hormone, the last anti-aging hormone to attract this much attention. Whereas hGH has to be injected twice a day, taking DHEA is as easy as popping a pill. And while a month's supply of human growth hormone costs hundreds of dollars, pharmacies can sell a two-months' supply of DHEA for under $30.

The Future of DHEA Therapy

Richard Podell, M.D., clinical professor of medicine at the University of Medicine and Dentistry of New Jersey–Robert Wood Johnson Medical School, says there have been three double-blind studies, two of which seem to show clinical improvement in middle-aged and older people when compared to placebos.[40]

"Results of my experience with DHEA in this group is that about twenty-five percent seem to improve," he says. "A few individuals have shown dramatic improvement that is unlikely to be a placebo effect because their symptoms have persisted for years.

These symptoms include fatigue, malaise, depression, loss of self-confidence, and general aches and pains.

"One of the most striking results was in a middle-aged man who tended to be depressed and have lack of self-confidence—the type of patient who would ordinarily be given an antidepressant like Prozac. He responded very well to DHEA. He said he felt better, more assertive, and calmer. Several women on DHEA said they felt better than they had in twenty years. They had suffered from fatigue, had frequent headaches and low-grade depression. We know that DHEA accumulates in the brain and modulates neurotransmitters."

Dr. Podell, who is the author of *Doctor, Why Am I So Tired?* (Fawcett), says his patients have their blood levels of DHEA tested, and if they are low, he gives men about fifty milligrams of DHEA that is compounded by a pharmacist and women about twenty-five milligrams.

"Women," he explained, "produce less DHEA."

The potential side effects, he has found, include mild acne and facial-hair growth.

Dr. Podell said that in the scientific literature, patients with autoimmune diseases such as lupus, rheumatoid arthritis, and thyroid inflammation have done well on DHEA. He said rheumatology reports, although not double-blind (in which neither doctors nor patients know which is the medication and which is the placebo), have concluded that 200-mg doses of DHEA are effective in reducing prednisone (a steroid medication with potentially severe side effects) and improving well-being. He said that he uses 25 to 50 mg in some of his patients with autoimmune disorders.

"Medical practitioners using DHEA today are typically prescribing three to thirty milligrams per day, although much larger doses are reportedly being given to patients with cancer, AIDS, and other serious conditions," he says.

The pharmaceutical industry has had little interest in putting its research funds or promotional dollars into DHEA itself, but its analogs (related compounds similar in structure but not identical in composition), which can be patented, are now intriguing pharmaceutical companies.

Arthur Schwartz, Ph.D., professor of microbiology at Temple University in Philadelphia, has been working on DHEA for more than twenty years, under National Institutes of Health grants.

"I first became interested in DHEA because it was lower in women with breast cancer," he says.[41]

He and his colleagues have developed an analog of DHEA, fluasterone, which does not have DHEA's masculinizing side effects in women such as raising cholesterol and increasing facial hair. He notes, "In animals we know that [DHEA] prevents cancer and counters diabetes and delays aging."

He said the first real DHEA pharmaceutical to treat the autoimmune disease lupus is now in Phase III (see Glossary) testing with a large number of patients.

"We expect the National Cancer Institute to begin trials with fluasterone in 1997 in women with ductal, in situ cancers of the breast, and in men with in situ cancers of the prostate," Dr. Schwartz says.

"These are cancers which are small, contained in one site, and are easily curable," he explains. The patients will be biopsied (a small tissue sample of the tumor is taken) before fluasterone treatment, and in two to four weeks, after treatment has begun, another biopsy will be done to see if the compound can prevent cancer growth.

Testing with fluasterone in patients with Type II diabetes is also scheduled to begin this year.

Dr. Schwartz notes, "We know that in high doses, androgens make diabetes worse, but in low doses it is very effective. This analog of DHEA has a dramatic therapeutic effect in diabetic animals. It has been tried in Phase I, where it is given to healthy people and has had no serious side effects. Phase II [see Glossary] studies in diabetic patients is the next step."

While Dr. Schwartz firmly believes that DHEA can delay aging, he points out that it is difficult to prove and will take years of observing biological markers of aging before it can be said that the hormone is effective. He has great hopes that it is effective against Type II diabetes, which usually occurs in middle age, and certain cancers that also occur in middle age and beyond.

Temple University has licensed fluasterone to a small pharmaceutical company, Aeson Therapeutics of Tucson, Arizona.

If fluasterone is effective against cancer and/or diabetes, Dr. Schwartz says, it will probably be about five years before it is approved for marketing.

What about the DHEA you can buy in your health food store or supermarket?

"It's a crazy situation," he says. "Nobody knows what dose is safe with those products. Chances are twenty-five milligrams will have no serious side effects, but two hundred milligrams might."

Drs. Regelson, Kalimi, and Loria of the University of Virginia Medical College note that in relation to DHEA as an anti-aging hormone, we have to consider its potential as a stress-modulating steroid. This is based on reports that suggest DHEA has a stress-mediated blocking action and thus helps prevent stress-induced injury to the central nervous system.[42] Studies at 90 mg per day and 40 mg per kilogram of weight per day showed improvement in mood and energy in one-third of the patients. This effect might be related to the high testosterone levels resulting from DHEA metabolism, as the researchers saw hirsutism and increased libido in several female patients.

This elevation in mood is not surprising since in Europe DHEA-S is marketed alone or combined with estrogen for post-menopausal depression. Italian researchers have studied DHEA in depression or fatigue syndromes with significant clinical results.

The National Institute on Aging's Dr. Bellino points out, "We don't know whether it is worth giving, but it is worth looking into. We have to await further research results to determine if there are positive health effects, and if so, what is the proper dosage and form of administration that will maximize DHEA benefits and minimize side effects. If it is beneficial, we want to know, and if it is dangerous, we want to know that, too."

THYMUS—BUILT-IN IMMUNITY

You don't have to be a scientist to be aware that, as the years go by, we are increasingly susceptible to infections such as influenza and pneumonia and to tumors. While there is tremendous interest in the adrenal glands' DHEA's part in stress, immunity, and aging, another endocrine gland—your thymus—plays an even bigger role in immunity. It is large in early childhood and starts downsizing at about eight or ten years, and by age twenty, it is only 5 to 10 percent of its original size. By fifty, just a scrap of the thymus remains.[43]

As late as 1961 virtually nothing was known about the thymus save that, in both humans and animals, it began to shrink early in life and often left only shreds of scar tissue by the time of sexual maturation. Then at the Chester Beatty Institute in England, Dr. Jacques F. A. P. Miller tried removing the thymus from newborn mice. For several weeks after their thymectomies, the baby mice seemed to thrive. But after that they fell ill and ultimately died of a disease marked by rapid weight loss and diarrhea. Postmortem examinations revealed an extreme depletion of the lymphocytes, or white blood corpuscles.

Rodents with their thymus glands removed became highly susceptible to spontaneous cancer. Among other symptoms they suffered were gray hair, thin and translucent skin, and loss of body fat. When autopsied, thymectomized mice had many different abnormalities including heart disease, widespread amyloid deposits, kidney disease, and destruction of the liver and pancreas. There were widespread tumors.

Apparently, the removal of the thymus may either allow growth of dormant malignant cells or allow bacterial or other infections to set off tumor growth.

But the elderly are burdened with a number of pathologic conditions that can impair their defenses. For example, diabetes is known to weaken immunity. Blood vessel disease reduces blood flow and compromises resistance to local infection and impairs wound healing.[44]

In human infants, it is believed the thymus produces white blood cells called lymphocytes, which are coded to recognize and protect the body's own tissue while they trigger an immune response against invaders. Later, other organs help out. Cells destined to become lymphocytes are born in bone marrow, the soft tissue in the hollow shafts of your long bones. Some of these cells, known as *stem cells,* migrate to the thymus and multiply and mature there into cells capable of producing an immune response. These cells are called *T cells.* Other white blood cells that appear to mature either in the bone marrow itself or in lymphoid organs other than the thymus are called *B cells.*

The T cells—which are so frequently counted in AIDS victims—do not secrete antibodies, but their help is essential for antibody production. Some T cells become helper T cells that turn on other T cells and B cells, which do produce antibodies. Other T cells become suppressor T cells, which turn off these cells. And still other T cells become killer T cells, which scavenge and kill enemy cells such as viruses.

T cells also secrete lymphokines, diverse and potent chemicals that can call into play many other cells and substances, including the elements of the inflammatory response. One class of lymphokines is interferon.

While the total number of T lymphocytes in the blood does

not change with age, only one-fifth to one-half the T cells from the thymus of an older person are able to proliferate and respond to an "enemy."

As for autoimmune diseases such as rheumatoid arthritis, lupus, and allergies, Sir F. MacFarlane Burnet, an English Nobel Prize winner, developed an immune theory of aging. He believed that the body becomes "allergic" to itself and self-destructs and noted three factors:

1. Aging in any species is genetically programmed as a result of evolution. The program is mediated essentially by a built-in metabolic clock.
2. Organs, or physiological systems, will differ widely in time needed to use up their quota of cells.
3. Many systems approach their limits, but that system, vital to life, that uses up its quota will be the chief secondary mediator of aging.

Everything points to the thymus-dependent (TD) immune system as the key system whose exhaustion is responsible for aging in mammals and probably other vertebrates. Remember that the thymus shrivels early in childhood. If the most essential function of the thymus system is to get rid of abnormal cells, then the system may control cancer and autoimmune diseases such as arthritis.

As pointed out before, the reason we humans die of so-called "old age" is usually because we are no longer immune to diseases. Although the cause of death may be listed as cancer or heart disease when autopsied, an older person may have had as many as twenty-five different diseases present, a situation similar to the one found in thymectomized mice.

If the thymus becomes less effective as we age and we lose our protection against viral disease, could it be possible that aging symptoms are caused by long-dormant viruses that come to life as our defenses wane? Those of us who have suffered from shingles (herpes zoster) after age fifty when the long-dormant chicken-pox virus we had as children reemerges to pain us can accept that premise. This theory also fits right into the observation that today's victims of parkinsonism are believed to be yesterday's victims of severe influenza infections. It would also explain why cancer is more prevalent in older age groups. With a thymus transplant in later years, we could then, if the theory is correct, have sufficient cells to fight off viruses.

If the shriveling of the thymus may account for the destruction of the body known as aging, would it be possible to take a piece of our thymus when we are young, freeze it, and give it back to us when we are older? This is just what was suggested by eminent immunologists at a science writers conference in 1971. And indeed, in 1972, two successful thymus transplants were performed in infants to give them immunity.

Since taking a piece of thymus from a healthy baby in the hopes of reimplanting it in middle or old age is not practical nor is transplanting a thymus from one person to another, modern scientists are concentrating on understanding and replenishing thymic hormones. Just recently, as this is being written, scientists have isolated hormones from the thymus, which they are now testing in humans.

Thymic humoral factor (THF), a natural peptide hormone isolated from calf thymus, reportedly increases the number of T lymphocytes and increases immunity in those with weakened or absent defenses.[45]

Thymopentin (Timunox) is a biologically active peptide that is similar to the thymic hormone thymopoietin. It is being developed for the treatment of HIV infections in people who have not yet shown the symptoms of AIDS.

Thymosin a-1, another thymic peptide, is being tested against chronic active hepatitis B and C, viral infections that affect the liver.[46] Naomi Judd, the country singer who had to give up touring because of chronic hepatitis, credits thymosin with saving her life.[47]

Thymostimulin (TP2) is a substance from the thymus that has been shown by Dutch researchers to have some slight promise against head and neck squamous-cell carcinoma, but the work is too early yet to draw definitive answers.[48]

A combination of **thymus humoral factor–gamma 2** and **alpha interferon** is being tested by researchers in London at Kings College School of Medicine in patients with chronic hepatitis B in whom all other therapies have failed. With the combination, three out of nine patients became negative for the hepatitis virus, and the Britons seem to think that the thymic hormone–interferon combination may be useful in treating chronic hepatitis B carriers.[49]

A report in the *International Journal of Immunopharmacology* by researchers from the University of South Florida lends rationality to all those who have been sucking on zinc lozenges to ward off colds or downing zinc tablets to improve their immunity. The Tampa researchers reported that zinc is incorporated into zinc-thymulin by the thymus gland, "a critical hormonal regulator of cellular immunity." The scientists from the Department of Internal Medicine at the university wrote that aged mice treated with zinc-thymulin had greatly increased response of the thymus cells to all stimuli, "indicating that treatment with zinc may have immunotherapeutic relevance, particularly in the aged and stressed organism."[50]

Ironically, not all our immune defenses are worn down. Our bone marrow stays pretty well intact. Aged bone marrow that is grafted into an irradiated animal has been found to repopulate the thymus as effectively as young bone marrow.[51] But as scientists learn more about our long-ignored, shrinking thymus gland, there is great hope that many of the ills that affect us, not only in old age but all through life, may be prevented.

If these thymus and DHEA products now in testing fulfill their promise, they may be used to combat the decline in immunity that occurs as we age and prevent many of the ills that we associate with it—maybe even keeping our hair from going gray.

3. Growth Hormones

Restoring Muscle, Bone, Fitness, and Well-Being

The boy who is much shorter than his peers and the girl who is a great deal taller than the tallest boys have serious social problems in our society. What makes them miserable is that their heights vary from what is considered the normal range for their age and sex. At the extreme of abnormal heights are the dwarfs and giants among us.

More than seventy years ago, a University of California at Berkeley professor found an answer to growth regulation. In an experiment with two dachshund puppies, Dr. Herbert Evans removed the dogs' pituitary glands. Nothing further was done to the first little dog, and it stopped growing. The second pup received injections of an extract of canine pituitary glands, and it continued to grow as if nothing had happened. At maturity, it was twice the size of its untreated litter mate.[1]

The secret of growth control, as many had suspected—and Dr. Evans proved—lies in the pituitary, a pea-sized gland situated in the center of the head behind the nose. The result of his experiment created a storm of enthusiasm. At last, short children and even dwarfs could be given pituitary extract and they would grow to normal height.

The solution was not that easy. Extracts of the pituitaries of dogs, sheep, or pigs were tried on dwarfed humans, but nothing happened. It became obvious that each species, including humans, produced its own unique growth stimulant.

Hopes for normal heights for too short humans were again raised in 1956 when Dr. Evans' disciple, Dr. Choh Hao Li, at the University of California's Hormone Research Laboratory, succeeded in isolating highly purified growth hormones from the pituitary glands of humans. Still, there were problems. It took more than one hundred pituitaries to provide enough hormone to treat a single patient. Trying to overcome this roadblock, U.S. and Canadian scientists harvested the pituitaries from corpses undergoing autopsy.[2]

This provided more growth hormone for undersized children, but another dreadful dilemma occurred. Some of the pituitary extracts contained Creutzfeldt-Jakob disease, more popularly known today as mad cow disease. It is a fatal, brain-destroying condition that usually occurs in the fifties or sixties. The infectious agent is a so-called slow virus that can be transmitted from animals and from human being to human being.[3]

Then, in 1981, researchers were able to produce in the laboratory a synthetic pituitary human growth hormone. While safe, it had only about 10 percent of the growth-producing potency of the natural one.[4]

There was then enough human growth hormone not only to administer to children with retarded growth, but also for researchers to study its function in adults. Lo and behold, it was found that human growth hormone has a profound effect on many body functions, including the metabolism of sugar, fats, and proteins. In the male, the growth hormone promotes the activity of the male hormone, androgen, and in the female, sex hormones function more effectively with hGH. Growth hormone also increases the production of disease-fighting antibodies.

On August 7, 1996, Eli Lilly and Company received FDA approval to market Humatrope, the first synthetic growth hormone for somatotropin deficiency syndrome (SDS) in adults. SDS adults may have a low output of growth hormone due to pituitary tumors, trauma, or other pituitary disorders, or they may have been treated for growth hormone deficiency as children. Adults with SDS suffer from metabolic disorders that affect their physical mobility, socialization, and energy levels, as well as their life expectancy. Some epidemiologic studies have suggested that adults with SDS are at greater risk of cardiovascular disease than adults without the disorders.[5] Doesn't it appear that the symptoms of SDS are similar to those in many aging adults?

The study of growth hormone and aging is one of the hottest areas of endocrine research today.

A part of the brain called the hypothalamus sits directly above the pituitary and gives it orders with two chemicals. **Growth hormone–releasing hormone (GHRH)** instructs the pituitary to *release* growth hormone, and **somatostatin** commands the pituitary to *inhibit* the release of growth hormone.

The pituitary-secreted **human growth hormone (hGH)** travels to the liver, its target organ, and induces production of yet another hormone, **somatomedin.** Somatomedin, in turn, acts on the ends of long bones, causing them to lengthen and a youngster's height to increase. In both children and adults, growth hormone also affects the nitrogen, fat, and water components of the body. Seriously ill or very aged people often go into negative nitrogen balance and lose protein and become weak and emaciated.

Problems can arise at various points in the hypothalamus-pituitary-liver interconnection. For example, overproduction of hGH due to a pituitary tumor can cause too much growth, resulting in gigantism. Conversely, if the hormone is produced in insufficient quantity or not at all, dwarfism results. Malnutrition, major organ disease, or chronic illness can also impede normal growth hormone production.

Even emotional deprivation can affect levels of growth hormone in the blood. Babies left in their cribs without the cuddling and love of someone who cares for them "fail to thrive," are undersized, and in extreme cases, die. Can isolation and loneliness in old age produce similar results? The interaction between growth and emotional deprivation is powerful!

Can supplementation of growth hormone maintain and restore strength and vitality while we pile up our birthdays?

Growth hormone peaks during puberty and falls by more than 50 percent by the time we reach thirty-three to forty years.

A number of researchers under grants from the National Institute on Aging are measuring the natural decline in growth hormones and how the drop affects the body. This is an effort to reenforce or refute those who say that the following aging effects can be reversed with supplemental human growth hormone or its stimulators:

- Fragile bones
- Loss of lean muscle
- Increased body fat
- Wrinkled skin
- Decrease in strength and endurance
- Loss of immune function
- Weakening of the heart

While these age-associated signs may be the result of many factors, no experts deny human growth hormone's importance in maintaining strength and immunity.

As pointed out before, your liver is the target organ of growth hormone from the pituitary gland in your head. Your liver produces a fairly recently discovered substance, *insulin-like growth factor (IGF)*, the level of which is regulated by how much growth hormone is available in your body.

Andrew Hoffman, M.D., and Steven A. Lieberman, M.D., of the Department of Medicine at Stanford University and the VA Medical Center, Palo Alto, California, and Gian Paolo Ceda from the Department of Geriatrics, University of Parma, Parma, Italy, considered growth hormone therapy in the elderly in *Psychoneuroendocrinology* in 1992. They wrote that because the growth hormone and IGF decline in aging, elderly individuals suffer from a syndrome that might be termed the *somatopause*. Lean body mass is diminished, fat deposits increase, and osteoporosis develops. Kidney function declines, and sleep disturbances are common. It is possible that GH and/or IGF-1 replacement therapy might reverse or prevent some of these "inevitable" sequelae of aging, they wrote. As long-term trials of GH therapy are initiated, however, it will also be important to measure the ability to think and behave in a careful and sophisticated manner, because it is likely that increased GH and/or IGF-1 levels will affect central nervous system functioning.[6]

As pointed out earlier in this chapter, the interconnection between emotions and growth hormone levels are strong, and this is a major reason some researchers believe that older people with low levels of growth hormone should be given supplementation. British researchers from United Medical and Dental Schools of Guy's and St. Thomas Hospital, London, England, for example, maintain, "Although many studies have focused on physical aspects of growth hormone deficiency and its treatment, there is evidence that psychological aspects may be at least as important, if not more important."[7] They wrote that validated patient questionnaires assessing psychological well-being have shown that GH-deficient adults perceive themselves as having significantly more physical and psychological health problems than control individuals matched for age, gender, social class, and geographical location.

The most striking abnormalities identified were poor energy, emotional lability, low mood, and social isolation. The British researchers reported, "The pathology behind these changes is unknown. Improvement in psychological well-being in response to GH treatment may be due to increased lean body and skeletal muscle mass; however, increased cerebral blood flow or perhaps a direct effect on the central nervous system are other possible mechanisms."

THE HEART AND GROWTH HORMONE

Patients with an enlarged heart have an organ that cannot beat as strongly as it should and that has increased stress on its walls. Most therapies today are directed to reducing the load on the heart, but do not specifically improve the underlying dysfunction.

What if the heart muscle could be made stronger and less dilated?

In a small study of seven patients, researchers from the University of Frederico II, in Naples, Italy, decided to see whether growth hormone could help. In patients born with deficiency of growth hormone, heart growth and function are impaired, and giving them growth hormone increases wall thickness and normalizes heart performance. Conversely, a long-term excess of growth hormone causes the heart to shrink and to beat too fast. Evidence is accumulating, they said, that growth hormone is a physiologic regulator of heart growth and performance.[8]

These observations gave the Italian researchers the idea to try growth hormone in the patients with enlarged hearts. In three months of treatment with genetically engineered (recombinant) growth hormone, the patients had their hearts reduced in size and beating stronger, and they felt much better during exercise and at rest.[9]

The University of Frederico doctors said their study was small and without placebo controls, but it should point the way to large clinical trials of longer duration to determine the effect of growth hormone in patients with enlarged hearts and other forms of heart failure.

Several researchers jumped in immediately to warn against the use of growth hormone in people with heart disease. They claimed, among other things, that long-term use of growth hormone may induce insulin resistance or overt diabetes and irregular heartbeat. The Italian authors answered the criticism by saying that the worry about insulin resistance or overt diabetes is well founded and that attempts are being made by combining growth hormone with insulin-like growth factor I. The incidence of irregular heartbeat occurred in a study using twice as much growth hormone as in their study.[10]

HOW MUCH GROWTH HORMONE IS ENOUGH?

The late Daniel Rudman of the Medical School of Wisconsin attracted worldwide attention when he reported in 1990 on an experiment in which HGH was injected into twenty-one healthy men ages sixty-one to eighty-one who produced little or no growth hormone. These volunteer subjects were given human growth hormone three times a week for six months to restore the circulating insulin-like growth factor (IGF) levels to the youthful range. IGF represents an indirect measurement of the circulating levels of growth hormone, since the secretion of growth hormone in the human brain is in a pulselike fashion and is difficult to measure during any period. In a few months, the men lost 14 percent of their body fat, gained 9 percent in lean body mass, and their skin increased in thickness by 7 percent.

Edmund Duthie, M.D., director of Geriatrics at Wisconsin, and his colleagues are continuing Dr. Rudman's study of human growth hormone with 288 men and women over sixty.

"We are looking to correlate levels of hGH with such things as the loss of muscle mass, increase in body fat, and the effect of exercise," Dr. Duthie said. "Testing the marker of hGH on many older people over a reasonable period of time will provide solid information on the clinical utility of hGH as well as on the risks associated with supplementation."

Dr. Mark L. Hartman, assistant professor of medicine, University of Virginia Health Sciences Center, Charlottesville, is a principal investigator leading a team under a National Institute on Aging grant to study the effects of growth hormone and physical training. The object of the study is to see whether the interventions, either together or separately, can reverse changes in body composition that come with decreased hormone levels and physical activities.

The study, which began with its first patients in 1993, has about forty participants at this writing. They are divided this way:

- One-third get no exercise training.
- One-third get supervised aerobic training four mornings a week.
- One-third are getting weight training three mornings a week.
- All inject themselves every night just under the skin with a substance. The human growth hormone is given in the fluid to some in each program, while plain fluid is given to the others. Neither the subjects nor the doctors know who is getting the real medication.

Dr. Hartman says that while those receiving the medication are unknown, all those in the exercise programs have shown marked improvement in muscle and strength.

The object of the study is to see whether growth hormone will increase the strength developed through exercise in older people, Dr. Hartman explains.

The study will go an extra year as will several others under the National Institute on Aging's grant because recruitment of those qualified to participate was difficult. They had to be healthy and active without ailments or medications that would obscure the treatment effect.

"We expected about a twenty to thirty percent dropout rate, but we had only three people leave," Dr. Hartman says. "One woman because she felt it took too much time to be in the clinical trial, and two others because of conditions not related to the program.

"One man, a former shop teacher, did have carpal tunnel syndrome, in which the nerve that travels through a tunnel formed by the wrist bones [carpals] becomes pinched when surrounding tissues swell. This side effect has been observed in patients taking growth hormone.

"The doctor who operated on him said the carpal tunnel syndrome had nothing to do with the program because he could see during surgery that the condition has been there for many years."

The man is back in the program, Dr. Hartman notes.

The University of Virginia researcher says the side effects have not been serious among the subjects because they start out with five micrograms per kilogram of weight, which they inject themselves, then go to ten and then fifteen micrograms.

"If they begin to show side effects on a higher dose, we go back to the lower dose," Dr. Hartman says.

He points out that the difference between his program and one of the others widely cited that showed no benefit from human growth hormone and exercise is that his subjects in his program inject themselves every day while in the other study they received just three injections a week.

"We have also monitored our patients' blood levels of human growth hormone every five to ten minutes for twenty-four hours," he notes.

His investigation, he says, is to see whether healthy older people—all of whom have lower human growth hormone than younger people—can benefit from supplemental hGH.

"We know that people who have pituitary tumors or other conditions that cause really low levels of hGH do benefit from supplemental amounts that restore their muscle strength and vitality," says Dr. Hartman.

Dr. Robert Schwartz, professor of medicine at the University of Washington School of Medicine, Division of Geriatric Medicine, Seattle, Washington, and his colleagues are working under a $1.25-million, five-year study funded by the National Institute on Aging.[11] Dr. Schwartz agrees many of the changes in body composition associated with aging are similar to those found in growth hormone deficiency. Elderly people have also been found to have significant abnormalities in several growth factor systems including growth hormone/insulin-like growth factors, and both male and female sex hormones.[12]

"This has led to intense interest in the clinical effects of growth factor supplementation in older individuals," he notes.

Dr. Schwartz is the lead researcher on a project studying growth hormone–releasing hormone (GHRH) and women. His group is using a synthetic form of GHRH, which is normally produced in the brain and helps control the amount of growth hormone the body produces. Dr. Schwartz says they decided not to give growth hormone directly because it has more potential side effects, and because they hope to stimulate older people's systems to start releasing growth hormone rather than rely on synthetic replacements.[13]

The decrease in growth hormone with age is believed to be due, in part, to decreased levels of GHRH. This is the substance that stimulates the pituitary gland to release growth hormone into the bloodstream. Supplementation of GHRH is one area of research that scientists believe may enable them to safely and efficiently increase human growth hormone production in the elderly.

"What we would like to determine is whether using a synthetic version of GHRH, a hormone that normally stimulates the body to produce its own growth hormone, will restart a system that has fallen asleep," Dr. Schwartz explains. "We need to find out realistically whether it has a place in treating frail people or preventing frailty."

The study will also look at whether stimulating the body's own growth hormone production along with an exercise program is more beneficial than either one separately.

"We want to know whether the body's own growth hormone can improve body composition, endurance, and strength, and whether any of these changes result in an improvement in women's ability to perform everyday activities such as carrying home a bag of groceries, making a bed, or climbing a set of stairs," Dr. Schwartz says.

Sixty-six women, sixty-two to eighty-four years old, are in his study. Compliance with the routine of self-administered injections is 90 to 97 percent, with only one dropout from the program, due to the routine's interference with her lifestyle.

A detailed health history and physical examination, including a strength and endurance-exercise tolerance test, were used to screen women for the study in 1993. The study began with a two-week weight stabilization diet. Participants were then randomly assigned to one of six groups:

- A group giving themselves injections of growth hormone–releasing hormone (GHRH).

- A group giving themselves inert injections.
- A group giving themselves GHRH injections and undergoing endurance training.
- A group giving themselves inert injections and undergoing endurance training.
- A group giving themselves GHRH and undergoing strength training.
- A group giving themselves inert injections and undergoing strength training.

Those in the exercise groups meet three times a week for six to twelve months. The study is blinded so that neither the participants nor the doctors involved know who is getting the GHRH and who is getting an inert substance. There have been few complaints of fluid retention and no documented cases of carpal tunnel syndrome, two common side effects of growth hormone therapy, Dr. Schwartz says.

Why only women in the study?

"Because they start out with less bone and muscle, live longer than men, and are more likely to become frail, so they would benefit most from this projective, if the results are positive," Dr. Schwartz explains.

One of the practical problems with human growth hormone should it be shown to be effective is that it must be injected.

Michael Thorner, M.B., D.Sc., director of the department of endocrinology at the University of Virginia, is studying an orally active compound, MK-677, from Merck Research Laboratories. MK-677 is not growth hormone itself but a synthetic version of a still mysterious chemical, called a secretogogue, that has been found to stimulate the production of growth hormone. While a lot of work has been done with secretogogue in animals, it was recently tested in seventeen men and fifteen women ages sixty-four to eighty-one. Their blood was sampled every twenty minutes for twenty-four hours, and after fourteen days of treatment, their blood was analyzed for growth hormone.[14]

"MK-677 caused growth hormone to be released in a pulsatile fashion in a pattern in the older participants similar to that of young people," Dr. Thorner says.

MK-677 is being investigated for growth hormone deficiency, enhanced recovery from injury—such as hip fracture—and to improve function in the elderly, according to researchers at Merck Laboratories.[15]

Marc Blackman, M.D., chief of the division of endocrinology and metabolism at Johns Hopkins–Bayview Medical Center, Baltimore, Maryland, is heading one of the largest anti-aging hormone investigations, the Growth Hormone Sex Steroid Intervention Study. All participants are healthy men and women over sixty-five. They have also been divided into four groups:

- Those receiving injections of human growth hormone and placebos substituted for the sex hormones.
- Women receiving estrogen-progesterone, and men testosterone, and a placebo instead of human growth hormone.
- Women receiving estrogen-progesterone, and the men testosterone, plus active human growth hormone.
- All in the group receive placebos.

Neither the investigators nor the participants know, as yet, who is getting what regimen. The Johns Hopkins endocrinologist says that there have been some mild side effects in some patients such as fluid retention and carpal tunnel syndrome. However, Dr. Blackman notes that there were few dropouts from the study, about 7 percent compared to an expected rate of more than 25 percent.[16]

Dr. Blackman said that the research is exciting: "What we are talking about is some very substantial improvements in our method of dealing with problems in aging persons such as thinning bones and weaker muscles. The ultimate upshot may be that replacement of human growth hormone and sex steroids in carefully selected older people can be given in a cost-effective manner."

The Johns Hopkins researcher warned, as did the others, that the studies are highly investigational, and that the effectiveness, safety, and cost of hormone supplementation must still be evaluated.

Danish researchers have already given uninterrupted growth hormone treatment in growth-hormone-deficient adults for three years. The patients were in their midtwenties and gave themselves injections of the hormone every day. Their exercise capacity and muscle strength were significantly increased, the Danes said, and the subjects' heart rates and blood pressures were stabilized. Their blood sugars remained normal, and at the end of the study no side effects were reported.[17]

Dr. Jens Jorgensen, who is at the Institute of Experimental Clinical Research in Aarhus, says, "We conclude that long-term GH replacement therapy in GH-deficient adults is associated with preserved beneficial effects on body composition and physical performance, resulting in a near normalization of several abnormal features and adding new merits to this treatment modality."[18]

The Danish patients were growth deficient and young.

A year later, Danish researchers reported on the short-term use of growth hormone in women between the ages of fifty-two and seventy-three. The patients underwent a week of treatment with either placebo or GH at dosages of 0.05, 0.10, or 0.20 IU/kg per day administered under the skin in the evening.[19] The growth hormone increased osteocalcin in the blood and also blood levels of collagen in dose-dependent fashion. These are two factors in bone health. With the lowest doses of growth hormone, the effects lasted just one to two weeks. With the highest doses, however, the effects lasted thirty days. Adverse effects were mainly related to fluid retention. They were dose dependent and rapidly reversible. The Aarhus University Hospital researchers concluded short-term GH treatment stimulates bone formation and bone resorption in postmenopausal women with thinning bones.

Not all the studies of aging and growth hormone are positive. A study done at Washington University School of Medicine in St. Louis, Missouri, found volunteers who received injections of human growth hormone and those who received injections of sterile water had the same benefits from exercise and no more. Kevin E. Yarasheski, Ph.D., and his coinvestigators, under a grant from the National Institutes of Health, studied twenty-three men who averaged sixty-seven years old. Fifteen received injections of sterile water. Eight were given injections of human growth hormone. All study participants lifted weights in a sixteen-week training program that consisted of high-intensity, low-repetition exercises. They exercised all major muscle groups in the four-days-a-week program, alternating each day between lower- and upper-body exercises. While the program helped build new muscle tissue and created new muscle protein, there was no difference between the two groups.[20]

Maxine Papadakis, M.D., and her colleagues at the University of California at San Francisco and the Department of Veterans Affairs Medical Center came to a similar conclusion. They recruited fifty-two healthy men over the age of sixty-nine with well-preserved functional ability but with low levels of growth hormone. They were given growth hormone—0.03 mg/kg of body weight—or a placebo three times a week for six months. Their body composition, knee and hand-grip muscle strength, endurance, and cognitive function were measured.[21]

The study's physical therapist assessed the participants' performance on nine physical functions. Participants were asked to write a prescribed sentence, transfer kidney beans using a tea-spoon, place a heavy book on a shelf, remove a jacket, pick up a penny from the floor, turn 360 degrees, walk a fifty-foot test course, and climb stairs to determine speed and the number of flights climbed before fatigue developed.

The men ranged from seventy to eighty-five with the mean age of seventy-five years. At six months, their bodies' lean mass had increased on average by 4.3 percent in the growth hormone group and had decreased by 0.1 percent in the placebo group. Fat mass decreased by an average of 13.1 percent in the growth hor-mone group and by 0.3 percent in the placebo group. No statisti-cally or clinically significant differences were reported between the groups in knee or hand-grip strength or in systemic endurance. However, the growth hormone group's score on the Mini-Mental Status Examination deteriorated by 0.4 whereas the placebo group's score improved by 0.2. Twenty-six of the men in the growth hormone group had forty-eight incidents of side effects. The most common was swelling of the legs and diffuse joint pain. Dose reduction was required in 26 percent of the growth hormone recipients and in none of the placebo group.

The California researchers concluded that the effective doses of growth hormone given for six months to healthy older men with well-preserved functional abilities increased lean tissue mass and decreased fat mass. Although body composition improved with growth hormone use, they said, functional ability did not improve and side effects occurred frequently.

The investigators conducting this study did point out that the small improvement in strength caused by growth hormone therapy had to be balanced against the side effects and cost of the drug. Moreover, they said, exercise alone in the elderly can achieve much greater increases in muscle strength. Whether higher-dose therapy would be more effective or whether longer-term therapy would prevent age-related decline in functional outcome is unknown, they said.

"Controlled studies in women and functionally impaired elderly persons would enhance our understanding of the clinical use of growth hormone," they advised.

Some researchers believe that growth hormone can be made more effective if it is given as the natural hormone is—in short bursts through the day—by pump administration. Others are experimenting with growth hormone–releasing factor and other substances that cause the body to produce more of its own growth hormone. And in the future, it may be possible to genetically alter human cells in a test tube to produce more hGH, then reimplant the cells in the body. This form of gene therapy has already been successful in animal studies.

Dr. Blackman of Johns Hopkins says the jury is not in on growth hormone, as yet. His study and two other big studies involving growth hormone sponsored by the National Institute on Aging have been extended for a sixth year.

He notes, "We cannot get hooked into making major conclusions on just one or two small studies. When the large, carefully controlled studies are completed, the pieces of the puzzle will fit together, and we will be able to say with certainty whether growth hormone does or doesn't improve muscle strength in the elderly."[22]

ADVERSE EFFECTS

Some studies have reported that as many as one-third of the elderly patients given growth hormone developed carpal tunnel syndrome, approximately 10 percent developed enlarged breasts, and a small percentage, high blood sugar.[23]

Growth hormone may be associated with cancer growth. Surgeons have removed pituitaries from women with breast cancer, leading to some remissions. In rats whose growth-hormone-producing pituitaries have been removed, injection of cancer-inducing substances and viruses seem to have no effect. But if the animals are then given growth hormone, cancer develops even though the hormone itself does not initiate cancer growth.

New studies, on the other hand, have found that aging men and advanced cancer patients can benefit from growth hormone treatments.

In Dr. Rudman's studies, the effect of growth hormone appeared to be temporary. The men saw their physiques return to fat after they stopped their injections. Some also experienced distressful side effects such as water retention, breast enlargement, and carpal tunnel syndrome. Some gained as much as twenty-three pounds of water weight, and even more serious, their blood sugar levels rose, increasing the risk for diabetes.

Side effects may be a matter of adjusting dosages.

COSTS AND AVAILABILITY

Gentech and Eli Lily developed hGH under the Orphan Drug Act of 1983, which offers pharmaceutical companies an incentive to develop drugs that treat fewer than two hundred thousand patients, a seven-year exclusive market. The parents of children who depend on it to grow to normal height pay $12,000 to $18,000 a year.[24]

A number of growth hormones on the market now are made by genetic engineering. They are sold under such names as Humatrope, Nutropin, Norditropin, and GenoTropin.

A form of human growth hormone, Serostim, was approved by the FDA in August 1996 for use in curbing the wasting effects of AIDS. The drug, manufactured by Serano Laboratories, Norwell, Massachusetts, which would originally have cost $75,000 a year, was lowered in price after pressure by AIDS activists.[25] Serostim helps fight the loss of weight and lean body mass that leads to death in many AIDS victims.

If growth hormone medications can be made in pill form, they should be less expensive, more easily administered, and perhaps easier to abuse.

It is estimated that at least a million Americans, half of them teenagers, are taking black-market physique boosters like hGH and steroids, which can cost up to $1,500 for a two-week supply. Although adolescent bodies produce plenty of the growth hormone, young bodybuilders believe they need more to make their muscles bulge.

Quite a number of persons on a quest for a youth-restoring elixir have gone to Mexico for shots of human growth hormone. HGH is available in the United States at research centers.

The Life Extension Institute, Palm Springs, California, offers complete hormone replacement with growth hormone as well as DHEA and melatonin and the male and female hormones. The initial consultation fee is $250. Pretreatment checks on blood levels of the various hormones run anywhere from $350 to $500 depending on how many hormones are checked. The cost of the human growth hormone is $200 per week. Discounts are available for prepayment, according to Dana A. Reisman, administrator.[26]

GROWTH HORMONE POTENTIAL

One therapy that is free and all the researchers studying growth hormone agree is beneficial to most older people is *exercise*. Aerobic and strength-training routines increase muscle and endurance. It's not new but it is still true.

What about growth hormone supplementation therapy for healthy aging adults?

"This is the most exciting time in endocrinology research," Dr. Thorner says. "We have more knowledge about hormones than in the past, and there are great advances in drug development. We are a step closer to understanding how secretogogue works. We are at the stage where we used to be with morphine for pain. We knew it worked, but we really didn't understand why."

Dr. Thorner, whose group is working under a grant from the National Institute of Diabetes, Digestive Disorders and Kidney Diseases, says there is a big question about whether the decline in growth hormone as we age is protective and similar to ovarian failure in menopause.[27]

"If you believe the way nature does things is right and you should accept [hormonal decline] as appropriate, then one should not interfere. If you accept estrogen replacement as the right thing to do, then you may believe that growth hormone replacement is appropriate. If you can take growth hormone by a pill rather than by injection, it will be better because, undoubtedly, it will have to be taken long term."

Dr. Thorner believes that estrogen replacement is correct, and he is studying the effect of estrogen on growth hormone. He also believes, however, that it remains to be shown whether growth hormone replacement will actually produce beneficial changes in body composition and function. He is certainly enthusiastic and hopeful about current research.

Dr. Thorner's colleague Dr. Hartman is also both enthusiastic and cautious:

"There is slowly accumulating evidence that human growth hormone supplementation does modify body composition, by lowering body fat, and it may also increase muscle mass. There is still the unsettled question whether that will result in health benefits—increased strength, better fitness, lower cholesterol, in the elderly."

In the next chapter you will learn about growth factors, those amazing substances in the blood that may aid growth hormone and other hormones to not only turn back the clock but have actually already proved their worth in growing new organs.

4. GROWTH FACTORS

Hormone Helpers
to Restore and Rejuvenate

Are you worried about wrinkles, age spots, thin, dry skin? Suppose you could grow youthful, new skin, made from your own cells. Science fiction? No, the procedure is being done right now to cover wounds and burns thanks to biotechnology and substances we make in our body called *growth factors* (*GFs*).

While you are reading this book, your hormones have growth factor helpers in your blood enabling you to ward off the many bacterial and viral infections, cancers, inflammations, and assorted ailments to which we, as human beings, are vulnerable. These GF "traffic controllers" stimulate and modulate cell activities.

The recent recognition that growth factors exist and the new ability to clone, imitate, or neutralize GFs will have a tremendous effect on how healthy you will be in the future; how you will be treated should you become ill; and how youthful your old age will be. They may even enable you to grow new organs or at least repair the ones you have damaged by age or illness. Fantastic? Skin and blood GFs are already on the market. Hundreds of others are being tested in humans to cure everything from cancer and AIDS to arthritis and wrinkles.

The idea that there is something in blood that can heal our

bodies is not new. At the beginning of the century, doctors took the colorless part of the blood, serum, from people who survived a disease and injected it into patients infected with the disease. The technique, *serotherapy,* sometimes worked, but it often caused side effects ranging from mild fever to fatal allergic reactions.

Serotherapy continued until the discovery in the 1940s of antibiotics that could quickly cure many infections. In the 1980s, however, scientists began to look again at serotherapy because antibiotics, while truly "wonder drugs," do have some major drawbacks. First of all, antibiotics are impotent against viruses; secondly, they have unwanted side effects; and thirdly, many germs have become resistant to them.

The existence of the substances in blood serum—now known as growth factors—that help fight disease was first suspected when it was noticed that blood serum could induce other cells to divide and multiply in laboratory dishes. In the 1950s, the first GF, nerve growth factor (NGF), a protein in blood that causes nerve cells to sprout, was identified. In the 1960s, a second GF, epidermal growth factor (EGF), was isolated. EGF stimulates the growth of epithelial cells that

- Form the outer layer of the skin.
- Line all the portions of the body that have contact with external air, such as the eyes, ears, and lungs.
- Specialize in secretions for the liver, kidneys, and urinary and reproductive tracts.

Epidermal growth factor has already proven its worth in the United States as an experimental treatment for burns and wounds. Two boys from Wyoming, who would ordinarily have died from third-degree burns over 90 percent of their bodies, were saved by EGF-produced skin.[1]

Organogenesis Inc. of Cambridge, Massachusetts, was expected as of this writing to soon have a skin product, Apligraf, approved by the FDA. It is made with the aid of EGF and will be used to cover wounds and burns.

Apligraf is one of a number of products called *reconstituted living skin equivalents*. It is made by putting skin cells on a plate where they develop through interactions between connective tissue cells and growth factors.

Researchers have also found that if another GF, *keratinocyte growth factor (KGF)*, in normal or wounded skin is deficient, the skin atrophies and thickens and there are abnormalities in the hair follicles. Upon skin injury, inhibition of KGF delays wound healing.[2]

And researchers are also testing another GF, *transforming growth factor–beta (TGF-b)*, found in embryos, to heal damaged tissue.[3]

Another company that is also producing "living skin" is Advanced Tissue Sciences, La Jolla, California. An ATS product currently in clinical trials for the treatment of diabetic ulcers is designed to be a permanent implant that can be used to build up the base of a deep wound. One of the reasons diabetics are prone to skin breakdown is that their skin cannot make adequate amounts of matrix proteins, according to Gail Naughton, chief operating officer of ATS. "What we are giving them is young, normal, healthy tissue … that grows into the human body, vascularizes, fills in the hole, and gives their own epidermis a healthy wound bed to grow over."[4]

"Skin is just the start," says Naughton. "You are going to see cartilage and bone, vascular tissue, GI tract tissue, and liver make very, very rapid progress."

In what is now called tissue engineering, researchers such as Prof. Linda G. Griffith-Cima, of MIT's Department of Chemical

Engineering, are manipulating individual cells to form complex, multidimensional structures that carry out the functions of normal tissue.[5]

Rice University in Houston, Texas, held its fourth annual course in tissue engineering research in 1996. At the meeting it was brought out that in addition to the two "living skin" products expected, at this writing, to be on the market soon, other areas that are rapidly advancing include

- Cartilage to reconstruct facial defects and knees. Tissue-engineered cartilage integrates smoothly into animals' joints, and clinical trials may have begun as you are reading this.
- Heart valves and blood vessels that grow along with the recipient. These have been implanted in animals and are expected to be tried in human patients within two years.
- Bone grown upon biodegradable polymer scaffolds, custom-shaped for each patient with the new bone eventually replacing the biodegradable polymer while maintaining the anatomically desired shape and mechanical properties. Bone has been grown in sheep, and preliminary results hold promise for future trials with patients.[6]
- Re-creating complex organs such as the liver, pancreas, and kidneys, which require different types of cells to interact to perform a variety of functions.

Researchers are also studying how these highly metabolic organs might, once developed, be integrated smoothly into a human so there is no interruption in nutrient and blood supply.

With tissue-engineered products expected to flood the market in three to five years, the FDA has established new guidelines for them.

Growth factors are making these tissue-engineered products

possible. More than one hundred growth factors have been identified since NGF and EGF were isolated, but it wasn't until recently
that genetic engineers were able to create tiny cell factories to produce enough GFs to use therapeutically. Cell factories are made
by combining two cells in the laboratory and manipulating their
genetic instructions so that the "combine" continually manufactures a desired cell.

In excess of 1,100 scientific papers have been presented
within the past two years on the subject of GFs, but the way hormones and growth factors work together is still being studied
intensively and enthusiastically by researchers around the world.
Scientists know that these chemical messengers selectively stimulate cell activities, which in turn affect critical events such as the
size and functioning of skeletal muscles. However, the pathway
from hormone to muscle is complex and still unmapped.

Take human growth hormone described in the previous
chapter:

- Growth hormone–releasing hormone (GHRH) from the brain
  stimulates the release of growth hormone (GH) from the pituitary gland.
- GH, in turn, stimulates the release of a substance primarily
  made in the liver, insulin-like growth hormone (IGF).
- IGF loops around and mediates many of the actions of GH
  from the pituitary.

When IGF enters the bloodstream, it seeks out special IGF receptors on the surface of various cells, including muscle cells.
Through these receptors it signals muscle cells to increase in size
and number. On June 24, 1996, the FDA granted patients with
amyotrophic lateral sclerosis (ALS) special early access to IGF
under the name Myotrophan. Between twenty thousand and thirty

thousand Americans suffer from ALS, also known as Lou Gehrig's disease. An illness of unknown cause, it involves muscular weakness and atrophy. It usually occurs after the age of forty and more frequently in men than women. It has been shown that IGF can slow the progress of the disease.

It has been determined that growth hormone and IGF both decrease significantly with advancing age.[7] The extent to which these age-related changes contribute to alterations in body composition and function remain to be elucidated.

Andrew Hoffman, M.D., and his colleagues at Stanford University Medical Center and the Veterans Hospital in Palo Alto, California, did a six-week study of twenty healthy women over sixty-five years of age.[8] They tested growth hormone and insulin-like growth factor (IGF). The latter, as pointed out before, is manufactured in the liver and regulates many of growth hormone's effects. The California investigators found that while total body weight remained constant, there was an increase of 2.5 pounds in lean body mass—muscle and bone—in women who received growth hormone and 8 pounds in those who received high-dose IGF-1.

Could IGF be the real agent in the maintenance of muscle and bone mass in women after menopause rather than growth hormone itself?

IGF has been found to affect bone and connective tissue. It is similar to growth hormone and it aids nitrogen retention, which is important in debilitating illness. It plays a part in turning boys and girls into men and women and in keeping bones strong. And it declines with age. Sixty-year-olds have 59 percent of the levels of IGF that twenty- to thirty-year-olds do; seventy-year-old men have 43 percent, and seventy-year-old women 54 percent; ninety-year-olds have only 29 percent.[9]

It has also been determined that bones contain IGF and

another GF, transforming growth factor–beta (TGF-b). The levels of both drop significantly from ages twenty to sixty. These GFs also interact with sex hormones, which are known to affect bone. TGF also aids wound healing and formation of cartilage.[10]

If IGF and TGF can help heal bones and wounds and EGF can regrow skin, perhaps nerve growth factor (NGF) can help heal brains.

GF BRAIN HEALERS

When you say, "You're getting on my nerves," to someone who is bothering you, you may be making a more scientific statement than you think. Increased NGF has been reported in both humans and animals after psychological and physical stress. Nerve growth factor has been known, for quite a while, for its actions on nerves and on the brain. Recent evidence, however, has shown high levels of NGF to be present in a variety of fluids after inflammatory and autoimmune responses, suggesting that NGF plays a part in immune reactions and stress.[11]

Lawrence R. Williams, Ph.D., a scientist in the Upjohn Company's Central Nervous System Diseases Research Unit, Kalamazoo, Michigan, has been working on the effect of this growth factor on the aging brain.

Although Alzheimer's disease, a degenerative brain disorder, was identified in 1906, its cause remains unknown. However, a growing body of research points to the degeneration of a specific group of nerve cells (cholinergic neurons) in the brain. These nerve cells supply acetylcholine, a chemical necessary for memory function and thought processing. In Alzheimer's, says Dr. Williams, cholinergic neurons atrophy and die.

"In experiments with young, brain-injured rats, untreated injured cholinergic cells atrophied and died," says Dr. Williams. "But injured NGF-treated cells lived and sprouted new extensions." His experiments show NGF reverses atrophy of nerve cells in the brains of aging rats. Furthermore, he said, others have demonstrated that old rats with memory impairment show behavioral improvement after treatment with NGF. Similar findings have also been reported in monkeys.[12]

"All of the animal data supports the hypothesis that the administration of NGF to Alzheimer's patients may improve symptoms of memory loss," Dr. Williams says.

Researchers at Johns Hopkins have been studying the effects of NGF in rats. Dr. A. L. Markowska and colleagues point out that it is well documented that NGF ameliorates age-related deficits in certain types of memory in rats.

"The issue of recent memory is of primary importance in the design of therapies for cognitive disorders because this type of memory is impaired in elderly humans and is severely affected early in the course of Alzheimer's disease," Dr. Markowska maintains.

Human NGF was infused over a period of two to four weeks into the brains of old rats. It showed no results after two weeks but produced memory power as efficient as that of young mice after four weeks.[13]

Studies are under way to determine the minimal effective dose of NGF and to find a better way to deliver it. Currently, NGF can only be effectively administered directly into the brain.

The problem in testing NGF is the blood-brain barrier. While substances pass easily from the bloodstream to cells in other parts of the body, the brain has a complex set of defenses that protect it from possible poisons. The blood-brain barrier includes physical barriers, such as tightly opposed cells in the walls of the blood vessels. Another defense is chemical—enzymes that act as gatekeepers, escorting only certain substances into the inner compartments.

Direct injection into the brain circumvents the barrier, but it is not very practical. Animal experiments with the NGF gene offer a possible solution. Researchers have found that the NGF gene can be incorporated into skin cells and then implanted in brains, where it has prevented the loss and degeneration of cholinergic neurons (see Glossary) involved in memory. Other researchers are looking at ways to package NGF and other growth factors with substances that can cross the blood-brain barrier, in effect smuggling these potential treatments into the brain.[14]

In addition to its potential with Alzheimer's patients, NGF is being tested to determine if it can help restore the function of some nerves that have been paralyzed by trauma or disease.

GFs May Help Repair the Human Brain

Fred Gage, Ph.D., professor, Laboratory of Genetics, the Salk Institute for Biological Studies, has found that adult nerve cells do retain the ability to regenerate, given the appropriate structures upon which to build. He has found in his laboratory that nonnerve tissue can act as a "scaffold," directing nerve cells to grow toward their target cells. In animals, he has harvested progenitor cells— basic cells from which other cells are formed—and with the addition of growth factors, he has stimulated the development of nerve cells. He has then grafted his creations back into the experimental host brain where they integrate into the brain in what appears to be a normal manner. Dr. Gage believes that similar principles apply in humans, and he looks to a future in which "damaged axons [nerves] can regenerate and progenitor cells can be directed to self-replace."[15]

University of Texas researchers harvested healthy cells from children undergoing brain surgery. The scientists then treated the cells in a laboratory dish with a mix of growth factors. Not only did the cells multiply, they sprouted interconnections and even began producing neurotransmitters.[16]

In preliminary experiments in which brain cells were implanted in rats, cells exposed to the growth factors survived while untreated cells did not. It may sound like science fiction, but the scientists are wondering whether brain cells could be programmed to perform specific functions. Perhaps with the right mix of growth factors, old human brains may one day be repaired.[17]

GFs May Help Restore Movement to the Paralyzed

Christopher Reeve, the actor paralyzed from the neck down, believes that nerve transplants aided by nerve growth factors will one day allow him to walk.[18] The man who once played Superman may be right. Research is in progress studying insulin-like growth factor (IGF) levels in spinal cord injury and paralysis. It has been determined that IGF is lower in such persons than normal, and the researchers who conducted the study at Mt. Sinai Medical Center in New York concluded that lack of physical activity in such patients results in depressed levels of human growth factor (HGF) and IGF and may be considered a state of premature aging.[19]

Another bit of evidence of the importance of IGF is that in the later years of life many polio survivors develop postpolio syndrome, manifested by progressive muscular weakness. Researchers at the Medical College of Wisconsin have shown that such victims have low IGF levels, and the older they were, the less they had. Further studies showed that low IGF levels were secondary to impaired growth hormone secretion. The Wisconsin investigators postulate that since low IGF levels resulting from growth hormone deficiency are known to be associated with weakness, muscle atrophy, and decrease in aerobic work capacity, it is postulated that low IGF levels have an adverse effect on aging polio survivors' nerve and muscle function, and that replacement therapy may improve their muscle function.[20]

Since insulin-like growth factor and human growth hormone

are both on the market, hopefully the next step will be to see if they may help spinal-cord-injured patients to regain some movement. Considering the success with skin and blood growth factors, it is certainly within the realm of possibility that growth factors will play a part in the rehabilitation of the paralyzed.

Growth Factor Inhibitors and the Paralyzed

Even newer than growth factors are growth factor inhibitors. These growth inhibitors are expected to have a wide range of uses, from stopping the growth of cancer and viruses to permitting the sprouting of new nerve cells.

Growth factor inhibitors may eventually be the keys that allow paralyzed limbs to move and brain cells to recover from damage. It has long been noted, for example, that nerve cells in the brain and spinal cord do not reconnect if they are cut or lost through injury. Dr. Martin Schwab and his colleagues at the University of Zurich believe that they may have made progress toward understanding why. Even when they flooded brain and spinal cord tissue in a dish with nerve growth factor, nothing happened. The Swiss researchers discovered that the covering of central-nervous-system nerves contains "neurite growth inhibitor," NI-35/250. When the investigators neutralized the inhibitor, the brain tissue in the dish began to sprout new spidery nerve extensions that carry messages between nerve cells. The Zurich investigators then neutralized NI-35/250 in rats who had injured spinal cord nerves. Within three weeks, the nerve fibers regenerated.[21] Earlier, Dr. Schwab and his associates found that the optic nerve in fish, which is able to regenerate after injury, contains a substance similar to nerve growth inhibitor but in very low amounts after injury, and they theorize that something happens when the fish eye is injured to add a growth factor and/or lower the growth inhibitor.[22]

Therefore, neutralizing growth inhibitors while adding nerve growth factor to damaged human nerves to make them regrow is within the realm of possibility in the not too distant future.

GFs AS IMMUNITY BOOSTERS

Aging and injury not only affect the skin and brain but the body's entire defense system. Another exciting GF category involves immunity boosters such as *colony-stimulating factors* (*CSFs*). These are a group of proteins produced by white blood cells that help defend us against invaders such as bacteria, cancer, and viruses. Schering-Plough Corporation, Kenilworth, New Jersey, and Sandoz Pharmaceuticals, East Hanover, New Jersey, are jointly developing *granulocyte macrophage colony-stimulating factor* (*GM-CSF*).

Eric Bonnem, M.D., director of oncology research at Schering-Plough, Kenilworth, New Jersey, says his company's research program is focused on GM-CSF's ability to stimulate cells that fight infections and tumors.

"The first promising area is as adjuvant [protective] therapy for chemotherapy patients," Dr. Bonnem explains. "In the United States today, aggressive chemotherapy is used for some advanced malignant tumors. The limitation to this therapy is often a life-threatening suppression of the white blood cell count caused by the cancer-killing agents. Worldwide trials with GM-CSF in lung cancer, lymphoma, and testicular cancer patients have shown that it increases white blood cells and is safe.

"This approach could enable these patients...to survive by maintaining their aggressive chemotherapy with GM-CSF."

Another area of investigation involves combining Schering's GM-CSF with Burroughs Wellcome's AIDS drug, AZT. As with cancer chemotherapy, one of the limitations of treatment with AZT is the suppression of white blood cells. Again, doctors have been able to continue AZT longer with GM-CSF.

GM-CSF, it is believed, could be of value in others who have weakened immune systems, such as the elderly or those who have life-threatening bacterial infections. Researchers are combining GM-CSF with current therapies such as antibiotics to see if the compound can save lives, shorten hospital stays, and decrease the use of antibiotics.

Other growth factors that are being tested as immunity boosters are the *interleukins 1, 2, 4,* and *6.*

The interleukins 1, 2, and 4 are growth factors that carry regulatory signals between blood-forming cells. The National Cancer Institute reports IL-1 activates T cells, special white blood cells that mature in the thymus gland and fight viruses and malignancies. IL-1 also stimulates bone marrow growth and has been shown to have direct antitumor effects on some human tumor cells grown from samples of melanoma (a potentially fatal skin cancer) and breast cancer tissue. In the laboratory, scientists also found that IL-1 can protect animals from lethal doses of total-body irradiation. IL-1 and IL-6 have, on the other hand, recently been reported to increase bone resorption—a factor in osteoporosis—in the elderly.[23]

Interleukin-2 was originally called T-cell growth factor because it spurred growth of T cells. According to the National Cancer Institute, now that there is a sufficient supply of IL-2, thanks to genetic engineering, more than fifty clinical trials are under way using IL-2 alone or in combination with other growth factors to treat advanced cancer and AIDS. In a report in July 1996 by National Institutes of Health researchers, self-administered injections of IL-2 dramatically increased the levels of infection-fighting T cells in patients with early HIV infection.[24]

IL-4, another interleukin, not only stimulates the growth of T cells but several other types of white blood cell defenders. It also "turns on" other growth factors, such as GM-CSF, that play a part in staving off infectious diseases. Scientists at Schering-Plough working with IL-4 believe that it also has a potential use in the treatment of AIDS and cancer patients, and it may help protect against the weakening of the immune system in the aging. Hoffmann-LaRoche has an IL-12 that has been reported to fight kidney cancer.

Schering has IL-4 in Phase II testing (in patients) for treatment of non-small-cell lung cancer. The company has IL-10 at the same phase for treatment of Crohn's disease and ulcerative colitis. Its IL-11 is on the market in Europe to treat side effects of cancer chemotherapy that causes blood clots.

BONE BUILDERS

Bones and beauty are the targets of yet another growth factor. *Fibroblast growth factor* (*FGF*) contributes to connective-tissue growth, tendons, bones, and skin. It also stimulates the formation of new blood vessels, which makes it possible for the body to supply nutrients to the new tissue.

PDGF is another GF originally found in platelets, the blood particles that are crucial to normal blood clotting. PDGF has been shown to cause tissue to grow and fill deep wounds.

PDGF has also been found to suppress the convulsions of epileptic mice, and this has led researchers to believe that lack of the substance may make mice and perhaps humans susceptible to convulsions.[26]

PDGF, however, may be an example of the dangers as well as the benefits of growth factors. In 1983 it was discovered that PDGF bore a resemblance to an oncogene, a gene that can cause cancer. PDGF is produced in abnormal quantities in some tumors, but it is not certain whether it is a cause or a result of the tumors. It may be that an oversupply of growth factors causes cancer, which after all, is an uncontrolled growth of cells.

BLOOD SUGAR, AGING, AND GFS

In younger people without diabetes, blood sugar levels usually rise 20 to 50 mg/dl of blood immediately after a meal and return to baseline two hours later. With aging, resistance to insulin gradually increases so that blood sugar rises to about 40 to 70 mg/dl in a sixty-year-old person after a meal and is much slower to return to baseline. Why? Five reasons have been suggested to explain the effects of aging on carbohydrate metabolism:

- Poor diet
- Lack of physical activity
- Decreased lean body mass in which to store the ingested carbohydrate
- Faulty insulin secretion
- Insulin opposition[27]

The exact cause of the changes of carbohydrate metabolism as we age is unknown, but among the clues is the effect of insulin-like growth factor (IGF).

In the summer of 1996, researchers at Stanford were beginning to test a potential treatment for Type I diabetes, the kind that requires insulin. Normally, a healthy pancreas responds to changes in blood sugar levels by secreting higher levels of insulin when needed, to help sugar enter cells so it can be used by the body as an energy source.

Type I diabetes, which affects about a million people in the United States, involves damaged cells in the pancreas that can no longer produce enough insulin to control blood sugar levels. The standard medical treatment includes insulin injections, usually about three a day.

Clinicians have treated diabetes with implanted pancreas tissue in the past, but because the tissue failed to flourish, the procedures were not entirely successful. The first attempt was in 1928, without success.

In the new strategy, Gregg A. Adams, M.D., and his colleagues at Stanford hope to overcome that problem by treating the newly implanted tissue with insulin-like growth factor 1 (IGF-1). In animal experiments, IGF-1 treatments helped pancreas cells proliferate and produce insulin.[28]

In the pilot study with ten patients, the California researchers implanted fetal pancreas tissue into the subjects' forearms, creating a row of about four implantations. The researchers are giving half the subjects IGF-1 injections and the other half none. Then they will compare the growth and function of the transplanted fetal pancreas cells in those who received IGF-1 and those who didn't. If it works, the patients with the IGF-1 who retain functioning pancreas cell implants will no longer have to take insulin, but they may have to take immunosuppressive drugs for the rest of their lives. That is why the first ten patients were selected from among diabetic kidney transplant patients who were already taking immunosuppressive drugs.

Scientists at the National Institutes of Health are recommending further studies to determine whether the addition of IGF to insulin replacement therapy may reduce the insulin requirement, maintain normal growth-hormone levels, and perhaps achieve better metabolic and anabolic balance in the treatment of insulin-dependent diabetes.[29] The information derived from those with diabetes may also point the way for IGF's use to restore a more youthful metabolism of sugar for older people without diabetes but who put on weight and lose muscle as they age.

OPENING UP ARTERIES WITHOUT SURGERY
With only one patient undergoing the treatment, worldwide interest was stirred up by a report in the British medical journal *Lancet.*

It concerned a seventy-year-old woman with severe blockage of the blood vessels in her legs.

Jeffrey M. Isner, M.D., of St. Elizabeth's Medical Center and Tufts University School of Medicine in Massachusetts, inserted a blood-vessel gene into the woman's leg arteries and added a growth factor, *vegF (vascular endothelial growth factor)* that allowed the woman to grow new blood vessels in her lower limbs. The new blood vessels were not sufficient to reverse the gangrene in her foot, and she had to have her leg amputated below the knee. However, the importance of the finding, researchers say, is that it shows the fundamental process in stimulating new blood vessel growth.[30]

Researchers are now looking for a vegF inhibitor because they believe the growth factor plays a part in eye disorders in diabetics. The growth of new, useless blood vessels to make up for lack of blood flow to the eye is a common cause of loss of vision in the adult diabetic.[31]

Another growth factor inhibitor, heparin sulfate (HS), affects smooth-muscle cells in the walls of blood vessels and may eventually lead to treatments for atherosclerosis (fat-cl-ogged arteies), complications after vascular surgery, miscarriages, heart attacks, and a rare lung disease in newborns, because all these conditions are characterized by excessive growth of smooth-muscle cells.[32]

Because GFs are so powerful and so much is unknown about them, the FDA, as an additional safety factor, is having growth factors tested in expensive primates rather than the more usual rats before they are tested in humans.

The therapeutic promise of growth factors, however, cannot be denied. Erythropoietin (EPO), for example, a growth factor that promotes red blood cell production, has been approved by the FDA and has been on the market for several years. It is being used to treat people on kidney dialysis and others suffering from chronic anemia.

An Ohio newspaper editor, who suffered anemia caused by dialysis treatment, needed weekly transfusions that haunted him with the fear of contracting AIDS. He felt so drained that he could barely drag himself to work. After two and a half years on EPO, the editor no longer needs transfusions, his anemia is under control, and he works out three times a week.

GROW NEW ORGANS TO REPLACE OLD ONES

Could a growth hormone or hormones be able to do what the so-called juvenile hormone in lower forms of life does? If so, we may all be able to grow new fingers, toes, and limbs if we need them. Creatures like the cockroach have the ability to regenerate missing limbs when young. However, once the cockroach grows old, it loses this ability.

In experiments at the University of Virginia, tiny holes were bored in the backs of young and old cockroaches, which were then fused so that their body fluids mixed. The legs of the old cockroaches were then amputated, and they promptly grew new ones. The juvenile hormone from the young cockroach enabled the old cockroaches to grow new legs. If scientists keep making the progress they are achieving with growth hormones, could regeneration be achieved in humans?

A University of Alabama scientist has even reported growing a new liver in a laboratory animal using a growth factor, *heparin-binding growth factor (HBGF-1)*. John Thompson and his colleagues at the National Institutes of Health implanted a small ball of angel-hair-like fabric used to line ski jackets next to a failing liver. The ball was first coated with HBGF-1 and other natural substances that stimulate cells to proliferate and to develop into blood vessels. In a matter of days cells began to grow, forming a bridge from the Gore-Tex to the liver. The bridge became a neo-organ or organoid. Healthy liver cells were injected into the organoid, developed a blood supply, and began to function normally.

"In essence, we grew the kind of cells necessary to take over the work of an ailing liver," Thompson said. "If we can do it with a liver, then I believe in the future we may be able to do the same with just about any other organs and arteries, including those attached to the heart."

The liver is the only internal organ in humans that can restore itself. University of California at San Francisco researchers and those at the San Francisco Veterans Administration Medical Center believe they may have a clue as to why—epidermal growth factor (EGF). Albert L. Jones, M.D., associate chief of staff for research and development at the Veterans Medical Center and professor of medicine and anatomy at UCSF, and his colleagues say that in rats with 70 percent of their liver removed, large concentrations of EGF appeared within hours in liver cells near the blood vessels supplying the tissue. In addition, EGF concentration was fifty-four times higher in the remaining liver cells just before they began to reproduce than in the liver cells of animals with intact livers.[33]

"One reason we are studying growth factor is that we foresee a time when whole livers wouldn't have to be transplanted," Jones says.

Although EGF is found in many body tissues, its range of functions is not completely clear. It appears to play a role in development of some tissues, including the lungs and teeth, and may stimulate growth of cells that line the intestines.

Researchers at the Syracuse Veterans Hospital believe that with proper electrical stimulation of cellular activity, the specific hormone would be released to enable limb regeneration in humans.

The frog, like the human, does not grow new limbs. Yet, frogs regenerate limb cells. When they were electrically stimulated, the cells dedifferentiated; that is, they changed back into cells capable of becoming something else, as if they were embryo cells.

If frog cells can dedifferentiate, then presumably so can human cells. By affecting the proper hormone balance with electricity, human cells that once had the ability to regenerate long ago in evolution may once again have it. Within twenty or thirty years, eminent researchers believe, we will be able to grow new digits and limbs if we need them.

Alan Goldhammer, director of technical affairs, Industrial Biotechnology Association (IBA), said, "When they were first discovered, it was thought growth factors had very small applications. We now know they have more apparent therapeutic usefulness than originally thought."

He said there are dozens of growth factors and some are already on the market—Cetus's Proleukin (interleukin-2), Schering's colony-stimulating factor (GM-CSF), and Immunex's colony-stimulating factor (G-CSF).

OTHER GROWTH FACTORS IN THE WORKS

Transforming growth factors (TGFs—alpha and beta and three beta versions) are among the newer growth factors discovered. The TGFs play a part in wound repair and help bones grow. They are active in blood vessel formation and inhibit tumors. Researchers are now theorizing that TGF may play a large part in age-related bone fragility.[34]

Angiogenesis growth factor (AGF) plays a role in the growth of blood vessels and may be useful in the treatment of cardiovascular diseases.

Megakaryocyte-stimulating factor (MSF) is believed to play a key role in stimulating the growth of platelets, elements in the blood that help initiate blood clotting. MSF may be effective in treating platelet deficiencies and as an adjunct to chemotherapy.

Glucagon-like peptide-2 (GLP-2). Researchers in Toronto

report that this substance stimulates the growth of the lining of the small intestine. According to the team leader, Dr. Daniel Drucker of the University of Toronto, "This finding may well result in major benefits for patients with severely compromised intestinal function, allowing treatment that will grow new cells in the lining of the small intestine." A human treatment may be available in three to four years.[35]

Heparin-binding growth factor (HBGF-1) is involved in the growth of blood vessels and smooth muscle cells. It may be important in tumor growth, wound healing, and the development of atherosclerosis (fat-blocked arteries).

Just as with estrogen or any other "anti-aging" therapy, there are potential side effects to growth factor use. Some physicians believe that colony-stimulating factors may play an important role in the development and progression of rheumatoid arthritis, an autoimmune disease, as pointed out before. They theorize that CSF regulation of the cells may be abnormal in rheumatoid patients and cause inflammation. Furthermore, slow-acting antirheumatic drugs may interfere with the activity of the growth factor network in the inflamed joints. The cause of rheumatoid arthritis and the action of antirheumatic drugs are unknown.[36] The hope is, of course, that when colony-stimulating factors are better understood, they can be used for therapy, when appropriate, and combated when they cause trouble.

IBA's Goldhammer points out that the understanding of growth factors and now growth factor inhibitors is really just beginning.

Barry Eppley, M.D., professor of plastic surgery at Indiana University Medical Center, has been investigating epidermal growth factor. He says it is being used in Europe in some skin-care lines. He said one major problem to overcome is that growth factors are active for only a short time.[37]

He says learning about GFs is similar to understanding blood clotting: "Once they figured out that it took one to thirteen factors to coagulate blood, they could develop drugs that prevented clotting. It is like a puzzle. We have many pieces, but there are still some missing. Once we put them all together, growth factors will be used for everything from healing, aging, and nerve regeneration to metabolic diseases."

In the meantime, a number of growth factor medications are on or approaching the market that will reverse some of the muscle and bone frailty of old age and possibly regenerate nerves in the brain and help the liver regrow.

GFs provide a whole new way of treating diseases. They control the development and specialization of cells. They have applications for almost any condition that may befall us, including AIDS, Alzheimer's, and cancer.

Because EGF has healing effects on the skin, there is some talk in the trade of putting it in cosmetics. But the Food and Drug Administration maintains that if a compound causes cellular changes, it is a drug, not a cosmetic, and must go through lengthy and expensive drug testing.

In the long term, whether or not GFs appear in your cosmetics, EGF will have many applications, including a big role in the regeneration of nerves and the healing of tendons, blood vessels, and corneal defects in the eye. If IGF can protect bones and build muscles, EGF can help heal skin, and perhaps nerve growth factor can help heal brains, then the possibilities of GF intervention in helping to restore old organs to a more youthful state are great.

A tremendous amount of research is now going on to develop growth factor products so that physicians will be able to prescribe them as easily as they do antibiotics and other medications.

5. THIN WITHIN—HORMONAL CONTROL OF WEIGHT AS THE YEARS GO BY

Estrogen, Leptin, Thyroid, and Insulin

Why is there such a thing as "middle-age spread" or a weak, flabby old age?

How is it that children can eat candy and ice cream and not gain weight while their parents may take a taste and put on pounds?

Who hasn't said, "I can't understand it. I don't eat that much and I still gain weight"?

New scientific discoveries are demonstrating that obesity has as much or more to do with inherited genes and body chemistry than with lack of willpower. Obesity is described as exceeding one's ideal weight by 20 percent. It is the most common nutritional disorder in Western societies and is recognized as a major metabolic disease throughout the world.

Everyone who has ever been on a diet knows how to lose weight, at least for a day or two. And every diet works, if we stay on it. But evidently, we are growing fatter, not thinner. Right now, we spend $30 billion a year in the United States in efforts to take off pounds. According to the National Institutes of Health, about a third of all women and a quarter of all men are trying to lose weight. The U.S. Centers for Disease Control and Prevention reports obesity is surging and that nearly one-third of Americans are at least 20 percent overweight. Carrying around that much extra poundage is a major risk factor for diabetes, heart disease, high blood pressure, stroke, sleep apnea, gallstones, some cancers, and forms of arthritis. On the other hand, can being about 10 percent underweight shorten or increase longevity?[1]

Experts now believe that anywhere from eight to thirty genes can contribute to weight problems. While no single gene causes obesity by itself, those who inherit several of them are more likely to have weight problems. But don't give up. New understanding of genetics and hormones is cutting through the "fat."

WHY WE GAIN WEIGHT IN MIDDLE AGE

Men may not go through menopause as women do, but older men just as older women don't burn as many calories as younger ones do, and their hormones may be the culprits.

Researchers at the Jean Mayer U.S. Department of Agriculture's Human Nutrition Research Center on Aging at Tufts, Boston, Massachusetts, fed an extra thousand calories a day for three weeks to a small group of men in their sixties and seventies and another group in their twenties. Both age groups had an increase in metabolic rate, but the older group had a smaller increase. The difference amounted to about eighty-seven calories a day, which the older group would store as fat if they didn't increase their exercise. That adds up to an extra 2.2 pounds per year or 22 pounds in a decade, the researchers estimated. The young men in the study reportedly automatically reduced their calorie intake after the overeating period, whereas the older guys continued to overeat.[2] Read on!

The lean body mass of an average male in his middle twenties is about 132.3 pounds; by the time he reaches seventy-five to eighty years of age, this falls to 105.84 pounds. During the same period, however, the fat content of his body doubles from 28 to 57.33 pounds. Loss of tissue occurs mainly from muscle, but some reduction occurs in the size of large organs such as the brain and liver. Similar changes occur in women, but to a lesser degree. This loss of active cells in our bodies reduces the need for energy-producing food.[3] Some believe the loss of these cells also accounts for the slow decline in metabolism as we age.

IS IT YOUR METABOLISM?

Metabolism, by definition, is the transforming of food into tissue and into energy for use in body growth, repair, and general function. Essentially all of the energy released from foods becomes heat. There, the metabolic rate is a measure of the heat produced by the body. We refer to it as "calories."

The average healthy person—if there is such a human being—in a quiet, resting state has a metabolic rate of about sixty to eighty calories per hour. However, multiple, interrelated factors can influence the metabolic rate, including exercise, ingestion of food, environmental and body temperatures, body surface area, sex, pregnancy, age, emotions, and state of nutrition.

And what paces our metabolism? Hormones! Hormones are made up of protein. Most experts believe that aging doesn't change our protein requirements, but some physical problems do. Surgery, acute illness, and some chronic diseases can increase the body's need for protein. Yet, results of national dietary surveys suggest that some older persons are not getting even the basic level of protein.[4] Protein not only creates body tissue—muscles, bones, hair, and nails—it also transports oxygen and carries the genetic code of life to all our cells. As if that weren't enough, protein is used by our bodies to manufacture antibodies, nerve cell messengers, and hormones! Insufficient protein can affect hormones as well as other body elements.

CHANGE OF LIFE AND WEIGHT

The influence of hormones upon weight can clearly be seen in the dramatic hormonal changes that occur during the "change of life." Menopause may cause more than just mood swings and night sweats; it also may lead to a "tire" around the middle.[5] Women going through menopause burn less fat and calories than younger women, whether they are active or at rest, and are also more prone to gaining fat and losing muscle, Baltimore researchers reported in the November 1, 1995, issue of the *Annals of Internal Medicine:* "There is something going on that is causing these women to get fat around their tummies."

The lead researcher, Dr. Eric T. Poehlman, of the Baltimore Veterans Affairs Medical Center, said, "If there is a target time to be concerned about exercising and dieting, it is when you are approaching or in menopause."

He and his colleagues periodically examined thirty-five healthy women ages forty-four to forty-eight for six years and found that although body weight remained the same, body composition changed. It is not known why menopause promotes fat gain, but this and other studies suggest that it may be linked to the dramatic drop in estrogen production that comes with menopause.

Some experts say the report is another piece of evidence that tips the scale in favor of estrogen-replacement therapy. Hormone therapy has already been shown to help ward off heart disease in postmenopausal women. And if it helps prevent weight gain—— a heart-disease risk factor—so much the better, proponents say. None of the women in the Baltimore study were on estrogen therapy.

William Andrews, M.D., past president of the American College of Obstetrics and Gynecology, commenting on the Baltimore study, said, "Modest doses of estrogen can cut the risk of weight gain. And very few women want to get fat around the middle. I think the logical thing to do for these women is to take estrogen, unless they are in a high-risk group for the diseases it may be linked to."

Charles Hammond, M.D., chairman of obstetrics and gynecology at Duke University Medical Center in Durham, North Carolina, was more cautious in his endorsement of estrogen and weight control: "This study is interesting, and although it suffers from small numbers of women in the study, it should be used as a palette for further studies on whether the pros outweigh the cons of estrogen therapy."

One of the first to examine the long-term use of estrogen and weight, Donna Kritz-Silverstein, Ph.D., and Elizabeth Barrett-Connor, M.D., of the University of California, San Diego, studied medical data from 671 women, aged sixty-five to ninety-four years, between 1972 and 1991. The researchers were looking for an independent association between hormone use, primarily estrogen, for fifteen years or more, and measures of obesity and body composition.[6] The women were classified as

- Never used hormone replacement therapy
- Used hormones intermittently for fifteen years or more
- Used hormones continuously for fifteen years or more

The researchers concluded, "After adjustment for age and baseline body mass index (BMI), there were no significant differences between any of the classifications on any follow-up measures of obesity, fat distribution, or body composition."

The UCSD investigators did find women using continuous hormone therapy were significantly leaner at the beginning, but after fifteen years of hormone replacement, they tended to catch up with the weight of nonusers.

Unlike previous, short-term studies, Drs. Kritz-Silverstein and Barrett-Connor said, this study adjusted for potentially confounding factors such as alcohol consumption, cigarette smoking, physical activity, and type of menopause (surgical or natural).

There were differences among the different classifications of women. Compared with those who never used hormone replacement therapy, continuous users had

- A significantly earlier age at menopause
- Significantly more postmenopausal years
- A tendency to have more regular strenuous or moderate exercise
- A drink of alcohol three or more times per week

Both continuous and intermittent hormone users were

- Significantly more likely to have had a surgical menopause than nonusers.
- More likely to report engaging in preventive behaviors to promote health since 1975 than nonusers.

Intermittent and current hormone users were

- Slightly but not significantly more likely to report decreasing dietary fat and salt, increasing daily exercise, and making other dietary changes since 1975.

The authors conclude, "The study confirms that hormone users tend to be leaner when first given estrogen and shows that neither long-term nor intermittent use explains or prevents the weight gain and central obesity commonly observed after menopause."

LEAPIN' LEPTIN

So women after menopause and men in their contemporary age group generally suffer from middle-age spread. The reasons why anyone gains weight—young or old, male or female—are not fully understood. No wonder, therefore, three reports in the July 28, 1995, issue of the journal *Science* about an obesity gene (ob) created a whirlwind of interest among scientists and consumers. The articles described the biological activity of the ob-produced hormone *leptin* by three independent teams. The gene had been identified by Rockefeller University researchers a year earlier. A strain of genetically obese mice that weighed three times as much as normal mice were found to have a mutation in the ob gene, and their fat cells did not produce ob hormone.

A research team from the Nutley, New Jersey, pharmaceutical company Hoffmann-LaRoche placed small amounts of leptin in the brains of obese and lean mice, and food intake was dramatically reduced and the mice lost weight. When the leptin was stopped, the mice regained the weight.

Researchers theorize leptin acts as a signal of how much fat is in the body to the brain's hypothalamus, which coordinates basic body functions such as eating. They believe differences in leptin fat production, resistance to leptin at its site of action, or a combination of the two could influence eating behaviors and metabolism to cause obesity or other nutritional abnormalities, such as diabetes.

Jeffrey Friedman, M.D., Ph.D., professor at Rockefeller University and an associate investigator with Howard Hughes Medical Institute (HHMI) says, "However, not all obese patients have increased levels, which suggest there may be important differences in the cause of obesity."

It is true the investigators found the amount of leptin in blood highly correlated to a person's percentage of body fat. However, the leptin level varied greatly from person to person. Women had significantly more leptin than men.

"The greater absolute leptin levels in women reflects that they have higher body fat content than men," Dr. Friedman reported.

Dieting can decrease leptin levels, and the higher the initial leptin level, the more it declines with dieting. Caution was sounded late in 1996 about leptin. Researchers at Israel's Weizmann Institute of Science found that a high level of leptin disrupts insulin response and may lead to diabetes and its complications.

YOUR SET POINT

The recent attention to genes and body chemistry has ironically returned attention to an older, controversial theory that we have a certain *set point* for weight and our body will defend that point against our efforts to reduce.

The set point mechanism—sometimes called the *adipostat*— is located in the brain. When changes in body fat and body weight are achieved by diet and exercise, a biological mechanism powerfully resists the changes and returns to the original weight. Leptin is a hormone that acts on the brain to lower food intake and fat buildup. As pointed out, one theory is that obesity may be associated with leptin resistance. To investigate the underlying mechanism, researchers at the University of Washington in Seattle measured the immune reaction to leptin levels in the blood and spinal fluid of fifty-three human subjects. They found a reduced efficiency of brain leptin delivery among obese individuals even though they had high blood leptin levels.[7]

Reduced sensitivity to leptin in some patients could explain why more leptin is found in obese people, the scientists note. "Some obese people may make leptin at a greater rate to compensate for a faulty signaling process or action," Dr. Friedman says.

"If resistance to leptin is partial, rather than complete, more leptin may be required for action."

Leptin's signaling ability may also help explain the high rates of regaining weight found among dieters, the investigators report. "After dieting, the levels of leptin drop, suggesting that less leptin is made and available to signal the brain," Friedman says. "This reduction may contribute to increased hunger and slower metabolism. If this is true, leptin therapy may help people maintain weight loss after dieting."

In addition, obesity may occur if genetic or environmental factors affect body chemistry after leptin acts, notes lead author Margarita Maffei, Ph.D., postdoctoral associate in Friedman's laboratory.

Shortly after revelation of the biological activity of leptin, Johns Hopkins University researchers reported in the August 10, 1995, issue of the *New England Journal of Medicine* about a gene mutation that causes a slowdown in metabolism. Those who have the faulty gene tend to grow potbellies and develop diabetes earlier in adulthood.

Art Campfield, Ph.D., of the Department of Metabolic Research, Hoffmann-LaRoche Pharmaceuticals, Nutley, New Jersey, whose company is developing drugs for obesity based on ob hormone, says it is believed no more than 50 percent of obesity is due to heredity, the rest being due to behavior.

Research has shown that on any given day, we may fluctuate between eating five hundred to a thousand calories more or less than needed.

"These new gene discoveries provide tools to open a black box," Dr. Campfield points out. "They will reveal new pathways for understanding the body's weight-control system."

Estrogen and leptin are two of the hormone players in today's obesity game receiving a great deal of press at this writing. Most of the research on diet, weight gain and loss, and aging, however, concerns the products of two other endocrine glands—the thyroid and pancreas. New information about them, however, may yield better therapy for both obesity and thinness, although the research is not as glamorous as gene and leptin research.

YOUR BUTTERFLY GLAND AND YOUR WEIGHT

In 1873, Sir William Withey Gull had observed among some women patients at Guy's Hospital a condition characterized by a dimming of mental faculties, some loss of memory, and a marked lowering of the basal metabolic rate evidenced by low body temperature and sensitivity to cold. The hair of these women tended to become dry and fall out, and the skin of their faces, arms, and legs grew puffy and swollen. Dr. Gull had no idea what caused this condition. But in 1888, another London physician, Sir Victor Horsley, demonstrated conclusively, by experimentally removing the thyroids of monkeys and other animals, that myxedema— as it had come to be called—was due to a loss of function of the thyroid gland. The thyroid gland, a butterfly-shaped body in your neck covering the sides and front of your windpipe, is a major governor of your metabolism—the rate at which your body fires burn.

Your thyroid gland emits a hormone, thyroxine (T4), under the control of thyroid-stimulating hormone produced by your pituitary gland. Thyroxine controls the rates at which chemical reactions occur in your body. Generally, the more thyroxine, the faster your body works. For this reason, thyroid hormones are sometimes used to treat obesity because they increase the loss of calories by speeding up metabolism. However, the hormones may also cause palpitations of the heart and other adverse side effects. Therefore, many doctors believe that the use of these agents should be limited to people who have thyroid deficiencies.

The Underactive Thyroid

Hypothyroidism (myxedema) is the underactivity of the thyroid gland. When it occurs, your thyroid gland produces only a small amount of thyroid hormone. Mild hypothyroidism increases with age and affects up to 15 percent of older women and 10 percent of older men.

Hypothyroidism can occur for no identifiable reason, or it can be caused by inflammation due to an autoimmune disease (see Glossary). With an underactive thyroid, your whole body slows down. Your feel continually tired and worn-out. Because body processes need less energy, you eat less but gain weight. You begin to feel cold more acutely. Your skin may be dry and thick. Your face may be puffy. Your voice may deepen and become hoarse. Mental tasks become difficult. You may have general aches and pains and move more slowly. Your heart may beat slowly and you may be constipated. All symptoms may be wrongly attributed to "just age."

Physicians often are quick to order blood tests because the disorder is so common in the aging. The diagnosis is difficult to make by just a physical exam, but easy when based on laboratory studies. The screening measures the level of thyroid-stimulating hormone (TSH) in the blood. The recommended policy by geriatric specialists, in fact, is that anyone over the age of sixty-five should automatically have a test for thyroid function.[8]

Like routine screenings for high blood pressure and breast cancer, screening for an underactive thyroid gland is cost-effective and should be part of periodic examinations for people over age thirty-five, especially women, a Johns Hopkins–led study suggests. The findings contradict recommendations by many physician groups that such thyroid screenings are unnecessary in the general population.[9]

"Early detection and treatment of mild thyroid failure can enhance the quality and even the duration of life," says Paul W.

Ladenson, M.D., lead author of the study and director of endocrinology and metabolism at Hopkins. "Our findings suggest that the health benefits are worth the costs, and that these screenings could be as safe, inexpensive, and effective as other common preventative tests in detecting early or hidden problems."

Researchers calculated the cost-effectiveness and impact on quality of life when people were screened every five years beginning at age thirty-five and received four decades of follow-up medication and care. These are comparable to screening costs for other disorders such as high blood pressure, breast cancer, and high blood cholesterol, with relief of symptoms, such as fatigue, weight gain, and depression.

Supplemental thyroid is one of the most prescribed medications in the United States. Replacement therapy is generally taken for life. Potential adverse reactions include chest pain, increased pulse rate, heart palpitations, hyperirritability, twitching, headache, excessive sweating, heat intolerance, insomnia, leg cramps, change in appetite, high blood pressure, fever, menstrual irregularities, and nervousness. It may increase the effects of anticoagulants and decrease the effects of insulin and oral diabetic medicines. Over-the-counter medications containing stimulants, such as many drugs used to treat coughs, colds, or allergies, may increase the side effects of thyroid medication.

If your favorite foods include cabbage, carrots, cauliflower, spinach, pears, peaches, brussels sprouts, and turnips, check with your physician. You may be reducing your thyroid hormone activity if you eat an excessive amount of those vegetables, which contain natural antithyroid substances.

The Overactive Thyroid

The overactive thyroid condition was relatively obscure until Pres. George Bush and his wife were diagnosed with it. Called Graves' disease, it can affect men and women at any stage of life, but there are seven women to every man who develops the condition, and it is most often found in people between ages twenty and forty. It is not as common as an underactive thyroid as the years go by, but it is not that unusual either.

If you have the classic or typical features of an overactive thyroid, you are probably nervous, have recently lost weight in spite of increased appetite, are having trouble sleeping, have a slight tremor in your fingers, and may be sweating more than usual. Again, all the symptoms may be attributed to "just age." Your doctor will examine your thyroid gland in your neck to feel if it is enlarged and listen to your heart to determine if the beat is too rapid. Your eyes will be checked to see if they bulge slightly.[10]

If you are older, you may not exhibit all of the classic symptoms of an overactive thyroid. Nervous symptoms evident in young people, such as hyperactivity, may not be present. You may, instead, feel tired, apathetic, or mildly depressed. You may not sweat too much, be intolerant to heat, have an increased appetite, or be irritable. You will, almost certainly, however, have eye symptoms.

The *Merck Manual of Geriatrics* states the overproduction of thyroid is even more of a masquerader than hypothyroidism in the elderly. The reason is that many of its symptoms may be similar to those often associated with aging, such as loss of appetite, heartburn, weight loss, exhaustion, depression, and bowel disturbances.[11]

The coincidence that both President Bush and his wife, Barbara, had the condition created quite a stir among thyroid specialists. Some suspected it might be due to a virus, but no infectious cause has yet been proven.[12]

There are curious and yet unexplained aspects of Graves' disease, particularly in the correlation between the symptoms and the severity of the thyroid condition. For instance, in some people,

relatively mild thyroid-hormone elevations can stimulate potentially dangerous heart-rhythm disturbances early in the disease.
Fortunately, once the thyroid condition is brought under control,
the cardiac symptoms quickly disappear.[13]

Although doctors have a good idea of what happens in the
thyroid gland itself as a result of Graves' disease, it is still not
known what triggers the assault by the immune system. People
can inherit a tendency to develop an overactive thyroid, but the
precipitating factors are still a mystery. Older people who have
high blood pressure or hardening of the arteries are believed to be
at greatest risk. Researchers are investigating various theories as
to what turns on the antibodies, but no solid evidence has been
presented to date.

On the bright side, an effective treatment exists for this common thyroid condition. In young and old, the level of thyroid hormone is measured, then adjusted with supplementation or
antithyroid drugs, such as propylthiouracil or methimazole, if it is
overabundant. Surgery is sometimes recommended.

Another endocrine gland besides the thyroid plays a big part
in how much you weigh—your pancreas.

DIABETES—THE SWEET AND BITTER DISEASE

The hormone-diet connection is nowhere more evident than in
adult onset diabetes. Of all mankind's afflictions, few have been
more common and more deadly than this hormone-deficiency disease, diabetes mellitus. At least two thousand years ago, Greek
physicians had learned to recognize its major symptoms: a wasting away of the flesh despite a raging thirst and a ravenous
appetite, and as the word *diabetes* indicates, a voiding of abnormally large quantities of urine. In the mid-1600s, the brilliant
British physician Thomas Willis provided his colleagues with an
even more definite method of reaching an early diagnosis: "Taste

thy patient's urine," he told them. "If it be sweet like honey, he will waste away, grow weak, fall into sleep, and die."

Two centuries later, another British physician, Dr. Richard Bright, noted at the autopsy table that the pancreatic glands of patients who had died of diabetes often contained numerous small crystals, or calculi. This observation led to the identification of the pancreas's involvement in the condition and then to the isolation of its hormone, insulin.

The pancreas is really two organs. It secretes enzymes, the workhorses of the cells, that help break food down into chemicals the body can use. As an endocrine gland, it puts out at least two hormones that regulate the metabolism of carbohydrates, plus other hormones with other functions. Most people have heard of only one pancreatic hormone that regulates blood sugar, insulin, but there is a second major one, glucagon.

Insulin and glucagon are put out by groups of cells in the pancreas called the *islets of Langerhans*. After a meal, when the level of sugar in your blood rises, the pancreas secretes insulin to reduce the amount, partly by helping to move sugar through cell walls and into the cells themselves. When the level of blood sugar drops below that needed by the brain and other tissues, the pancreas secretes glucagon. That hormone increases the amount of sugar in the blood by mobilizing supplies of it from the liver. It also helps inform your brain that you are hungry. Glucagon is used therapeutically to treat low blood sugar and is also used in insulin-shock therapy for depression and for severe insulin-induced low blood sugar during diabetic therapy.

INSULIN DEFICIENCY

The development of obesity often results from the secretion of insulin from the pancreas and of steroid hormones from the adrenal gland, and by a decreased rate of secretion of growth hormones from the pituitary. However, this does not mean that such abnormalities are the cause of obesity, since they often disappear when the body weight is reduced to normal. Nevertheless, once the abnormalities are established, they may make it difficult to lose weight.[14]

Diabetes mellitus, on the other hand, is a disorder of carbohydrate metabolism that occurs because the body either secretes too little insulin or is incapable of using the insulin that it does secrete.

There are two main types of the disease. In Type I diabetes, which is also called insulin-dependent or juvenile-onset diabetes, the pancreas produces little insulin. This type usually appears suddenly in childhood and is the more serious of the two kinds.

In Type II diabetes, non-insulin-dependent or maturity-onset diabetes, the pancreas may produce normal amounts of insulin, but for some reason the body cannot use it to metabolize carbohydrates.

The two types have in common the fact that much of the sugar in the body cannot get into the cells and so accumulates in the blood and is excreted in the urine. One eventual result of uncontrolled diabetes may be a disturbance of fat metabolism. This abnormality can lead to sudden coma and death and over a long period may be responsible for the complications of diabetes—prematurely clogged arteries, strokes, kidney disease, and eye damage. In other words, it speeds up those conditions we associate with old age.

A National Institutes of Health (NIH) Consensus Development Conference on Diet and Exercise in Type II Diabetes concluded that obesity and aging promote the development of the disease in susceptible individuals.[15] The prevalence of Type II diabetes increases steadily from the fourth decade. Individuals who are twenty to thirty pounds overweight are clearly at risk, and the risk accelerates with increased body weight. Excess upper-body fat appears to be associated more with diabetes than lower-body fat. Individuals with a family history of non-insulin-dependent diabetes may develop the disease when they have only a modest excess of body fat.

Extensive studies demonstrate that obesity is characterized by insulin resistance. In the obese nondiabetic individual, the principal target issues for insulin—liver, skeletal muscle, and fatty tissue—do not respond appropriately to those levels of the hormone found in normal-weight individuals. The obese nondiabetic person can compensate for this impairment of hormone action by secreting increased amounts of insulin. Weight reduction in these nondiabetic individuals leads to reversal of insulin resistance and the return to a normal pattern of insulin secretion.

Pancreatic beta-cell dysfunction and insulin resistance are the cardinal pathologies of Type II diabetes. Both these cellular alterations may be genetically determined. Although insulin resistance is present in the nonobese patient with Type II, associated obesity further aggravates the severity of impaired hormone action. Aging is associated with an increased accumulation of abdominal fat, glucose intolerance, and insulin resistance. Researchers from the Department of Medicine, University of Maryland School of Medicine, and the Baltimore Veterans Affairs Medical Center tested in a group of obese middle-aged and older men the theory that diet-induced weight loss would reduce not only belly fat but improve glucose tolerance and insulin action.[16] Oral glucose tolerance tests were performed before the regimen started and again after nine months of diet-induced weight loss in thirty-five men with an average age of around sixty. They were compared to a similar group not participating in the diet. Those on the regimen lost about twenty to twenty-four pounds, had an 8 percent reduction in waist circumference, and had a 2 percent reduction in waist-to-hip ratio. Weight loss improved glucose tolerance in all the subjects in the study, and nine of the men achieved normal glucose tolerance.

Those who did not participate showed no improvement, and in fact, their intolerance increased. Weight loss in the obese diabetic, as in the nondiabetic, ameliorates insulin resistance, and usually there is an accompanying improvement in carbohydrate tolerance.

Frequently, high blood sugar is reduced when a low-calorie diet is employed even before there is much weight loss. Furthermore, some studies have also shown modest improvement in pancreatic beta-cell function when the blood sugar is lowered by diet or other means. The NIH expert panel said that although the cellular alterations responsible for Type II diabetes are poorly understood, you can do something about it yourself. You can arm yourself with knowledge about diet and exercise and reduce your weight.

THE AGE FACTOR AND WEIGHT

There is, no matter what any of us do, a gradually progressive decrease in glucose tolerance that occurs with age—but there is no significant change in fasting blood sugar. The decrease in glucose tolerance is particularly evident in the nonfasting state after a high-sugar-drink challenge is given.[17]

In younger subjects without diabetes, blood sugar levels usually rise to 20 to 50 mg/dl immediately after a meal and return to baseline two hours later. With aging, resistance to insulin gradually increases so that after a meal blood sugar concentrations rise about 5 mg/dl more with each decade. Fasting blood sugar concentrations, however, change little during aging—1 to 2 mg/dl every ten years.

Five mechanisms have been proposed to explain the effect of aging on carbohydrate metabolism:

1. Poor diet
2. Physical inactivity

3. Decreased amounts of lean body mass in which to store the ingested carbohydrate
4. Impairment of insulin secretion
5. Insulin antagonism

Although low carbohydrate intake and physical inactivity contribute to glucose intolerance, these factors do not entirely explain the age-associated deterioration of carbohydrate metabolism. Similarly, although lean body mass definitely diminishes with age, this tissue redistribution cannot explain age-related changes in carbohydrate metabolism. Diminished insulin secretion does not cause the glucose intolerance of aging. Almost all studies in which the insulin response to various stimuli has been assessed in aging have shown normal or even increased insulin concentration in older individuals.

In contrast, insulin antagonism has consistently been shown to be associated with aging, especially in persons around sixty. The mechanism, however, remains a mystery.[18]

Arizona University researchers in Tuscon are studying glucagon's part in diabetes, and their work may give further clues to why Type II diabetes may develop in adulthood. Drs. Victor Hruby and Bassem Azizeh and their colleagues theorize that insulin abnormalities first limit diabetics' utilization of blood sugar and then excess levels of glucagon boost their blood sugar levels even higher.[19] They have set out to prove this theory and potentially treat diabetes by designing compounds to block the action of glucagon. They recently developed glucagon analogs that lowered blood glucose levels in diabetic animals by as much as 40 percent—without administering insulin. Drugs developed from these glucagon analogs could potentially be used instead of insulin to control diabetics' blood sugar levels. But Dr. Hruby says his group will also test these compounds in conjunction with insulin, checking for synergistic effects. One potential application where this could be especially handy is in the treatment of ketoacidosis, a life-threatening condition in which diabetics go into shock. Insulin alone can't turn ketoacidosis around fast enough, and patients may end up in the hospital for an extended period or may even die. Hruby says, "But we're hoping we can turn it around much faster with these glucagon analogs."

About 25 percent of diabetics take insulin, 50 percent receive oral medications that stimulate the pancreas to emit insulin, and the remaining 25 percent are controlled by diet alone.[20]

The effort to control weight with medications takes three basic tacks:

1. Reduce appetite with anorexic agents.
2. Promote loss of water through urination with diuretics.
3. Increase the proportion of food energy lost as heat with thyroid or other compounds that speed metabolism.

EXERCISE, HORMONES, AND WEIGHT

Exercise, as has been promoted in recent years, does indeed have an impact on weight and on diabetes. An interesting study conducted among the islanders of Mauritius in the southwest Indian Ocean made this clear. The islanders don't have to work hard to survive and laze around the island enjoying themselves. Researchers from the University of Pittsburgh Graduate School of Public Health went to Mauritius because the islanders had an unusually high prevalence of maturity-onset diabetes (non-insulin-dependent diabetes mellitus).[21] The high rates were found among all ethnic groups including Indians, those of African origin, and Chinese. The researchers found a high correlation between physical activity and blood sugar, especially in the middle-aged inhabitants. The less they exercised, the more likely they were to have diabetes. This was true even though body mass, waist-hip ratio, age, and family history were considered.

MALE HORMONE AND OBESE WOMEN

Women with weight problems have often accused men of causing them to overeat. Well, now some women may be able to blame their excess poundage and even their diabetes on male hormones. Researchers at the Medical College of Wisconsin have shown that sex hormones influence the type and distribution of fat cells in premenopausal women. Male hormones, they say, also appear to determine a woman's risk of getting diabetes, regardless of the presence of obesity.

Ahmed Kissebah, Ph.D., M.D., professor of medicine at the Medical College of Wisconsin, found that a "subtle increase in the male-to-female sex-hormone ratio in women who take in more calories than they expend results in enlarged fat cells that are deposited from the waist up."[22]

A corresponding decrease in the male-to-female hormone ratio results in an increase in the number of normal-size fat cells that are deposited below the waist.

An increase in male sex hormones also contributes to insulin resistance, Dr. Kissebah maintains. This stage precedes diabetes and is associated with a higher risk of heart disease.

To determine the role of male-to-female hormone ratios in obesity in women, Dr. Kissebah's volunteers were eighty healthy women between the ages of twenty-five and forty. Their weight ranged from normal to more than twice their ideal body weight. Of the eighty participants, twenty-two were upper-body obese, twelve lower-body obese, twenty-seven intermediate with overall distribution of fat, and nineteen nonobese. None of the eighty had any clinical evidence of hormonal abnormality or metabolic disorder.

Blood samples from the study subjects were measured for levels of male and female sex hormones and fat distribution. The upper-body obese had the highest male-to-female hormone ratio.

This higher ratio was accompanied by an increase in blood sugar and insulin levels, suggesting, the researcher says, that women with upper-body obesity need more insulin to remove blood sugar from the body.

Dr. Kissebah suggests that "early detection of an increase in the male-female sex-hormone ratio should be a signal to women that they are at a higher risk for diabetes. Active measures should be taken to keep their weight down."

WHEN YOU WEIGH TOO LITTLE

In animal studies, dietary restrictions have increased longevity. This may also be true in human beings. But what about being significantly underweight?

The study of underweight is as sparse as middle-aged people who are too thin in our society. Researchers from the Departments of Preventive Medicine and Clinical Epidemiology at Harvard Medical School did assess the condition in a meta-analysis (see Glossary) of major prospective studies.[23] They found that obvious (clinical) or subtle (subclinical) illness can reduce body weight, thus artificially increasing the mortality attributable to lower weights. The observation that excess mortality among underweight individuals tends to occur most often early in follow-up while overweight-related mortality is delayed suggests that underlying illness (perhaps enhanced by the higher prevalence of smoking) is contributory. The Harvard researchers noted that in a prospective study of ninety-one patients with involuntary weight reductions, 25 percent died during the first years after the first visit, supporting the ominous implications of unintended weight loss.

The Harvard investigators noted that major studies of relative weight and mortality have not addressed simultaneously the biases resulting from lack of control for cigarette smoking, inappropriate adjustment for the biologic effects of obesity, and failure to eliminate artifacts of disease-induced weight loss.

Contrary to the suggestions of several investigators, the Boston investigators maintain, it is clear that overall mortality is lower at weights that are at least 10 percent lower than U.S. average weights, and that there is no convincing evidence for a protective effect of weights above average.

"There is certainly some point at which extremely low relative weight is deleterious, such as in eating disorders," the Harvard researchers note, and conclude, "Since the mortality hazards of moderate obesity are less than those associated with tobacco use, cigarette smokers should focus on their efforts on terminating their smoking habit before attempting to control their weight."

YOUR MIND AND YOUR WEIGHT

Women know that the hormonal shifts of menstruation and pregnancy are often behind certain cravings. Studies show that many women eat chocolate, for example, right before and during their periods.

For the most part, food aversions are learned, usually from feeling nauseated or getting sick after eating something—even if the food wasn't the cause of the queasiness.

Sarah Leibowitz, Ph.D., of Rockefeller University, New York City, says we do have specific appetites for things. We do like salt and carbohydrates. These cravings are controlled through the brain. Reducing levels of serotonin—the brain chemical messenger involved in temperature regulation, mood, and sleep—suppresses the appetite for carbohydrates, she says, and she and her colleagues have found that if they inject a certain brain chemical, neuropeptide Y, into the brain of animals, they crave carbohydrates. She and other researchers at the forefront of brain and eating behavior agree that the interaction is complex.[24]

The flavor cravings of some obese people can be due to their association of taste with a medicinal effect. Persons who crave sweets are often addicted to what they describe as a "sugar rush." Sugar turns on the sympathetic nervous system, and carbohydrates can increase mood-elevating levels of serotonin in the brain. The result is diminished pain sensitivity and decreased appetite.

Food is connected with many significant events in our lives. It can be an expression of love and friendship and an important feature of holiday and other celebrations. Food and our emotions are strongly connected. When food becomes a means of coping with anger, depression, and feelings of inadequacy and loneliness, the pattern becomes addictive and dangerous.

Duke University researcher Theodore Pappas, M.D., assistant professor of surgery, believes that eating is in part controlled by two separate hormones: first, neuropeptide Y, which is a brain hormone that triggers the desire to eat and drives eating behavior during the meal, as the Rockefeller University researchers found; second, cholecystokinin (CCK), which is released when food is swallowed and the stomach inflates. This second brain hormone causes cessation of eating behavior and therefore "satiety."[25]

Dr. Pappas believes that these hormonal signals are not effective in the morbidly obese: "These people continue to eat even through their stomachs are filled. The signals that normally stop appetite and promote satiety are not working. Our research suggests that there is a hormonal imbalance: either they do not have enough of the CCK off-switch, or have an excess of the on-switch, neuropeptide Y. The bottom line is that what was once considered a societal problem is very likely a medical problem with a biochemical basis."

Still another brain hormone was reported to play a part in appetite, eating, and obesity by researchers at the Joslin Diabetes Center and Brigham and Women's Hospital in Boston. A compound, melanin-concentrating hormone (MCH), is found, they said, in higher levels in the brains of obese mice than in lean mice. When MCH was injected into normal mice, the animals consumed about twice as many calories as usual.[26]

While the function of MCH is unknown, it is produced in the hypothalamus, that area of the brain believed to be in control of weight regulation. Leptin, mentioned earlier in this chapter, is produced by fat cells and may, the Boston researchers believe, signal the brain to release MCH or other appetite-stimulating or appetite-suppressing compounds.

SUMMING UP THE HORMONE-WEIGHT CONNECTION

Emotions, food, behavior, and hormones are all interconnected. How much one affects the others is the subject of much study, many theories, and every person's experiences. It is difficult to separate hormone output from other factors in weight control. It is known that hormone secretion may be altered by such elements as the climate, diet, emotions, and the amount of body fat. For example, the development of obesity often results from the secretion of insulin from the pancreas and of steroid hormones from the adrenal gland, and from decreased secretion of growth hormones from the pituitary. However, this does not mean that such abnormalities are the cause of obesity, since they often disappear when the body weight is reduced to normal. Nevertheless, once the abnormalities are established, they may make it difficult to lose weight. Weight gain, furthermore, is only one of the consequences of passing years, and the complicated role that hormones play is far from completely understood. As more information is gathered, however, chances are it will be easier to lose weight and, what is more important, maintain normal weight in the not too distant future.

6. MELATONIN

The Time of Your Life

In 1729, an astronomer by trade, Jean Jacques d'Ortous de Mairan, reported an interesting plant phenomenon to the French Royal Academy of Sciences. He observed the leaf movements of a mimosa that opened its leaves during the day and folded them at night. When he moved the mimosa to a place where the sun could not reach it, he found the plant still opened its leaves during the day and folded them for the entire night. De Mairan is credited with being the first to report of the persistence of circadian (about twenty-four hour) rhythm in the absence of environmental time cues such as light and dark.[1]

We humans also have inner clocks that keep our bodies on an approximate twenty-four-hour schedule. They also time how fast we age. Can these inner clocks be deliberately stopped or reset?

One of the major hopes to repair an off-beat timer or to slow or reverse what we call aging involves our hormones. They are the pacers that transmit information from one body site to another. Rather than releasing their substances into the bloodstream continuously, most endocrine glands appear to secrete only intermittently. As a result, hormone levels in the body consist of a series of highs during emitting episodes, and lows during the turn-off period. The endocrine glands and their hormones are wonderfully synchronized.[2]

Most vital biological processes exhibit a circadian rhythm including our metabolism, body temperature, neurotransmitters (nerve messengers), gastrointestinal activity and digestion, immune system activity, liver function, blood pressure, blood constituents, and of course, concentrations of hormones. In fact, it is difficult to find any of our bodily functions that are devoid of such a rhythm. The timing effect on body processes has many knowns and unknowns, but some manifestations are fascinating. For example:

- Women go into labor most often between 1:30 and 2:30 A.M. and least frequently about midday.
- Heart attacks are twice as likely to occur between 8 and 10 A.M. as between 6 and 8 P.M.
- Dental pain and stomach ulcers are worse at night than during the day.
- Migraine headaches, hay fever, rheumatoid arthritis, and the crushing chest pain of angina all usually occur and are more severe during the morning.
- Eating a meal a day of two thousand calories results in a weight loss when eaten as breakfast but produces a weight gain as supper.
- Aspirin stays in the body longer when taken at 7 A.M. than when taken at 7 P.M.
- The senses of hearing, taste, and smell are more acute at 3 A.M. and fall off rapidly to a low at 6 A.M., then rise to another peak between 5 and 7 P.M.
- The allergic react more strongly to allergens at around 11 P.M., while antihistamine drugs have the greatest impact in the morning.[3]

Doctors can actually measure the ebb and flow caused by hormonal timers. For example, they gave people one liter of water to drink at 10 A.M. and measured their urine flow, which was 16 ml/min. When they gave the same people the identical amount of fluid at 3 P.M., their urine flow never exceeded 8 ml/min. The physicians concluded that the response of the kidneys to hormones that affect function differs markedly depending on the time of day.[4]

The variation in daily rhythm is well known and well used in women during their reproductive years. In the latter half of the menstrual cycle after ovulation has occurred, the mean temperature becomes elevated. A woman who wishes to become pregnant (or to avoid conception) by the rhythm method must take her temperature every day around the same hour to determine when ovulation is taking place.

This delicate hormone-influenced fertility timing was dramatically displayed when the first attempts at in vitro fertilization ("test tube" babies) were made. The pioneers of the technique, Dr. Patrick Steptoe and Dr. Robert G. Edwards, were at first successful in only four women out of seventy-nine. In all four, the ovum implantation was performed between 10 P.M. and midnight—a 100 percent success at this single two-hour period of the day. Just think about when most babies are conceived naturally and it makes sense.

The recognition of the importance of body rhythms has given birth to a new and growing specialty—chronopharmacology. This means timing medications so they are most effective. There are circadian variations in the way drugs are absorbed, metabolized, distributed through the body, and excreted. The uptake of oral drugs may be affected by circadian variations in the stomach and intestines. Some drugs such as Valium or antidepressants concentrate more rapidly when given early in the morning than when given in the evening. Researchers theorized that if an asthmatic took his oral steroid drugs—which keep airways open—in the afternoon instead of the morning or evening, they would have peak levels of the drug in the blood at night when they are most vulnerable to an asthma attack. The theory proved true. One asthma patient who tried it was able to lower her daily dose of steroids from forty milligrams to ten milligrams, and thus reduce the drug's side effects, merely by taking the drug at 3 P.M. instead of 8 A.M.[5]

There is now an emphasis on giving cancer chemotherapy when malignant cells are most vulnerable and the patient is not.

In one study, mice were injected with a toxin. Eighty-five percent died when injected at one time of day, but only 20 percent died when the same dose was injected twelve hours later. In another study, one group of mice was given chemotherapy drugs in doses that varied over time, and a second group was given the drugs at a continuous level. Both groups received the same total amount of the drugs, but about 95 percent of the mice in the first group survived compared with only 70 percent in the second group.[6]

In still other animal research, investigators at the University of Arkansas for Medical Sciences and at Stanford University have been able to lower the toxic side effects of drugs used to treat leukemia by varying dosages according to circadian rhythms. Most cancer cells, they found, lose their rhythmicity. They determined the time when the normal cells were not as sensitive and administered the treatment at that time to shield healthy tissue.[7]

So the body clocks that tick every day to time body functions according to the twenty-four-hour cycle are paced by hormones. How about the body clocks or clock that controls our aging and how long we are going to live? What can be done to repair or reverse a faulty inner clock?

In keeping with the earth's rotation, our twenty-four-hour timers are influenced by external as well as internal cues. Light, for example, is a great "clock winder." After passing through our eye's retina (light-color receptors), light signals a part of our brain known as the hypothalamus, which oversees our emotions, movement, and eating. Less than the size of a peanut and weighing a quarter of an ounce, this small area also influences our blood pressure, sexual behavior, and sleep. Within the hypothalamus is a tiny pinhead-sized group of cells known as the *suprachiasmatic nucleus*—believed to be the master biological clock.

Many today maintain one of the most powerful hormone "timers" is melatonin. It is secreted by the pineal gland, a tiny bulge deep in the brain behind the forehead. Once thought of as a vestigial "third eye," the pineal's function had been overlooked. Today, however, researchers are actively studying this endocrine gland because its hormone melatonin

- Is produced only at night.
- Is high in youth and declines in middle and old age.
- Has been found to prolong life in animal studies.
- Is capable of altering the sleep-wake cycle.

There is no doubt that melatonin, like other hormones, has a biorhythm and may itself affect the ticking of the twenty-four-hour clock. It may also affect the length-of-life clock. To delineate where in the brain melatonin acts, a team of Harvard investigators used radioactive-labeled melatonin to study its target site in the brain. It localized consistently in the *suprachiasmatic nucleus,* the master biological clock.[8]

Melatonin is secreted in a rhythm that is highly dependent on the light-dark cycle.[9] Dubbed the Dracula hormone by some, melatonin in your blood is low through the day, begins to rise in the early evening before the onset of sleep, reaches its peak at about midnight or soon thereafter, and then declines, whether or not you sleep. The duration of melatonin secretion depends on the duration of the darkness, so that twenty-four-hour melatonin secretion is greater during the winter than during the summer. Exposure to light at night inhibits melatonin secretion in a dose-dependent fashion: the brighter the light, the greater the decrease in plasma melatonin concentration. On the other hand, exposure to darkness during the day does not increase melatonin emission.

At the time and immediately after a change to night-shift work or travel across time zones, melatonin output is desynchronized and contributes to that hangoverlike fatigue we call jet lag.[10]

Prolonged nocturnal melatonin secretion is believed responsible for the winter-induced regression in sex hormone secretion in animals; the administration of melatonin not only inhibits reproductive activity in mature animals but also delays sexual maturation in immature ones. The hormone is the timekeeper that triggers seasonal breeding. Since humans do not breed seasonally, the role of melatonin has long been obscure, and biologists suspected it was just an evolutionary relic.

Are the reproductive lives of humans also affected by melatonin? The occurrence of both delayed and precocious puberty in children with tumors in the pineal region has led to study of the role of melatonin in human reproductive physiology. Among patients with precocious or delayed puberty, however, nocturnal melatonin secretion is usually appropriate for their age. Women living in Finland secrete more melatonin during the winter than during the summer, but the length of their menstrual cycle does not differ. Nocturnal melatonin secretion is also slightly increased in women with exercise-induced absence of menses or with the eating disorder anorexia nervosa. Men with underdeveloped sexual organs also have increased melatonin.[11]

Nighttime plasma melatonin concentrations are highest in children one to three years old and adolescent eight- to fifteen-year-olds and decline gradually thereafter so that adults fifty to seventy years of age produce only about 10 to 14 percent of the melatonin that young children do. The drop is believed due in part to the pineal gland's unusual propensity to calcify. Pineal calcification can be detected by computed tomography (CT) scans in young children, and it's found in about 30 percent of persons ten to twenty years old and 80 percent of persons over thirty. The more pineal calcification, the less melatonin secretion in adult humans.[12]

The pineal is probably the only source of circulating melatonin, since melatonin all but disappears from the blood after the pineal is removed. Much is unknown about how it goes about its job, but some researchers believe that it would make a good marker of brain aging in humans.[13]

The idea that melatonin can slow aging is primarily based on animal studies done in the 1980s.[14] The discovery that melatonin functions as an age-controlling hormone in mammals was demonstrated by two sets of researchers. In 1979, Dr. Dillman and his coworkers gave epithalamin to rats, which, as they later showed, stimulates melatonin production.[15] Twelve years later Walter Pierpaoli, M.D., Ph.D., coauthor of the best-seller *The Melatonin Miracle* (Pocket Books, 1995), and colleagues at the Biancalana-Masera Foundation for the Aged in Ancona, Italy, directly administered melatonin to mice. Both Dr. Dillman's and Dr. Pierpaoli's groups observed a surprising 25 percent increase of life span in mice, postponing old age.

The National Institute on Aging's Dr. Monjan says sound scientific data demonstrates melatonin's relationship to circadian rhythms and sleep. He said NIA has not yet received any applications to study melatonin's life extension potential.[16]

HYPE OR HELP?

The lack of knowledge about all the effects of melatonin hasn't stopped it from being embraced by the lay public. Melatonin, sold in health-food stores nationwide in America, is being touted as a cure-all for everything from sleep disorders and jet lag to cancer and AIDS. By some accounts, melatonin can prevent or cure diabetes, cataracts, Alzheimer's disease, schizophrenia, and epilepsy. Other proponents have claimed that the hormone can reverse aging and energize a lackluster sex life.

Many people are swallowing everything publicized about the product of the pineal.

Andrew Monjan, Ph.D., chief of the Neurobiology of Aging Branch at the National Institute on Aging, who oversees the distribution of research grants for melatonin, says, "The claims that melatonin is a powerful antioxidant occur in tissue culture systems at levels much higher than produced in the body."[17]

Russell Reiter, Ph.D., coauthor of *Melatonin: Your Body's Natural Wonder Drug* (Bantam), writes that high doses of melatonin can kill free radicals, highly reactive molecules generated when a cell "burns" its food with oxygen to fuel life processes.

Free radicals act as "loose cannons," rolling around damaging cells. This damage is thought to be a first step in cancer development. Antioxidants can suppress free-radical cell damage.

Dr. Reiter, a neuroendocrinologist and longtime melatonin researcher at the University of Texas Health Sciences Center in San Antonio, injected rats with a toxic substance known to cause cancer by unleashing large amounts of free radicals, which damage the DNA, the genetic makeup of cells. Dr. Reiter's measurements found that the rats receiving melatonin had 1 percent as much DNA damage as was found in the rats not given melatonin.

Dr. Reiter concludes that DNA damage in the unprotected rats would presumably have produced liver cancer if the experiment had continued. He also did experiments involving human white blood cells in a dish. The melatonin again seemed to protect against radiation damage to the cells.

Production of oxygen free radicals also contributes to the

generalized biological wear and tear we refer to as aging. Rats treated with melatonin developed varying degrees of resistance to cancer-causing chemicals. Melatonin-treated rodents have acquired resistance to cataracts, cloudy spots that form in the lenses of aging eyes as a result of oxidation.[18]

In an earlier experiment, Dr. Vladimir M. Dillman, a Russian researcher, and coworkers isolated a biologically active pineal extract (epithalamin) in rats. They found that giving rats melatonin did not affect the rate of tumor incidence but did delay onset of tumors by 257 days. Female rats given pineal extract over twenty months, furthermore, lived 10 to 25 percent longer and had far fewer estrus abnormalities than those not given it.[19]

Whether or not melatonin prolongs life is still uncertain, but as NIA's Dr. Monjan points out, there is evidence that melatonin does affect sleep.

SLEEP-WAKE CYCLE

A good night's sleep can make you look and feel younger. How does melatonin affect the sleep-wake cycle? Before its full impact can be understood, we need to know why we sleep and why we wake up. Our body clocks still keep ticking while we sleep. Every ninety minutes or so, our brains cycle through different stages of sleep.

In stages one and two, often called light sleep, brain activity begins to slow down as we move from wakefulness to slumber.

In stages three and four, sleep deepens as our brain waves slow down.

The fifth sleep stage is characterized by REM (rapid eye movement) and occurs four or five times a night with a high level of brain activity. During REM sleep, brain waves are similar to those of wakefulness—fast and of low voltage—and autonomic activities such as heart rate and blood pressure are irregular.

Breathing and heart rates speed up and there are mild involuntary muscle jerks. Most of our dreaming occurs during REM sleep. REM-sleep deprivation has been associated with impaired memory of past events and acquisition of new memory.[20]

Non-REM sleep, the dreamless period, is considered the stage during which our bodies are rejuvenated. Brain waves are slow and of high voltage; heart rate and blood pressure are low and regular.[21]

Sleep is defined as the biological and behavioral state in which humans are normally quiet and relatively unresponsive to external stimuli, traditionally thought of as the time when we end our day of work and activity. What happens when we don't get enough sleep?[22] Disrupted or diminished sleep can

- Impair concentration, judgment, and reaction time, making our ability to perform even simple tasks more difficult and increasing the chance of having an accident at home, at work, or while driving.
- Block creativity.
- Deplete the number of important disease-fighting immune cells in the blood.
- Be linked to chronic aches and pains, such as arthritis and fibromyalgia (muscle pain and fatigue).

More than seventy sleep disorders are identified by the American Sleep Disorders Association, and the causes can be internal or external.[23] When we refer to a sleep problem, most of us think of the trouble falling asleep we call *insomnia*. There are basically three types:

- **Transient**—lasts just a few days.
- **Short-term insomnia**—lasts several days or weeks.

- **Long-term or chronic insomnia**—lasts longer than a few weeks.[24]

There are many causes of insomnia:

- Medications can disrupt sleep.
- Poor sleep habits, such as napping intermittently throughout the day and keeping rooms darkened so that the brain actually becomes confused as to whether it is night or day.
- Depression and anxiety disorders both cause insomnia, and patients suffering from chronic insomnia should always undergo psychiatric evaluation. Insomnia and depression have long been closely linked. In fact, improved sleep often precedes improvement of mood in patients taking antidepressant medications.[25]

It has been estimated that over half of the 29 million people now over the age of sixty-five in the United States experience some disruption of sleep. Although changes in circadian rhythms have been viewed as part of normal aging, new information indicates that many of these disturbances may be related to pathological processes that are associated with aging.[26]

Can a hormone reset the clock and induce more natural sleep?

AGING AND SLEEP

Sleep patterns vary considerably according to age. Infants usually have unpredictable nighttime sleep and frequent daytime naps. Young adults average one long nocturnal period with one awakening and no daytime nap. Older adults' sleeping patterns evolve into something much like infants. By the age of sixty, the number of awakenings per night averages about six. The light sleep (stage one) of a sixty-year-old is about two and a half times greater than a young adult's while the REM sleep and stage two sleep show lit-tle change. Deep sleep (stage four) diminishes markedly in the av-erage sixty-year-old, by about 15 percent to 30 percent.[27]

Researchers have found that in many people over sixty-five the sleep-wake cycle shifts. Consequently, unlike younger people, who typically have trouble falling asleep at night and awakening early in the morning, older individuals tend to have trouble stay-ing awake in the evening and sleeping past 3 A.M. or 4 A.M.

Not all older individuals show marked changes in their sleep patterns, however. For example, although the average number of awakenings was six, about 20 percent had no awakenings, while others had ten or more. In an intensive study of sixteen fifty-year-old males, four had no deep sleep while three had the amount of stage four sleep present in thirty-year-olds.[28]

Most studies have reflected a difference between men and women in aging and sleep. The sleep of women is, in general, more resistant to age changes. One study found the sleep of sixty-year-old women essentially ten years "younger" than that of men of the same age.[29]

Although older people's ability to sleep may change, their need for sufficient, restful sleep does not. Most people need at least seven and a half hours to function adequately and be fully alert the next day, but some may need as little as five while others need nine to ten hours.

In a study conducted at the National Institute of Mental Health in 1993, people given the opportunity to sleep as long as they could averaged about eight and a half hours of sleep per night. The subjects in this study, who normally averaged a little over seven hours of sleep a night, said that the extra sleep made them feel more energetic, happier, and less fatigued.[30]

About 3.5 percent of U.S. workers work night shifts, averag-ing about six hours of sleep a day when on that shift. They must sleep in the daytime, when the body is programmed for wakefulness. Daytime sleep is less restful than sleep at night.

If you consider how much our ancestors without electricity slept—nine to seven hours—*it may be that we are shortening the time our natural circadian rhythm mandates we should sleep.* Overloaded personal schedules and a twenty-four-hour-a-day economy are causing chronic sleep deprivation for millions of Americans, according to leading sleep experts.[31]

Sleep patterns vary. Ask yourself if you are

- A lark, a person who is full of energy upon awakening, while others—often a mate—are still trying to become conscious.
- An owl, a person who comes alive as darkness falls and others get ready for bed.
- An insomniac who awakens in the wee hours and tosses and turns.
- A SAD individual (seasonal affective disorder), who feels blue in the winter.
- A frequent traveler suffering from jet lag.
- A night shift worker who is out of sync when the weekend or vacations arrive.
- A wintertime weight gainer who, like a bear, is prepared to hibernate and then lose the fat in summer.
- A lover who is sexier in the spring.
- An after-lunch sluggard.

All the above are the results of your biological clock. Can your timing be reset with melatonin or by changes in behavior?

MELATONIN AND SWEET SLEEP

Is melatonin the sleep hormone? Pineal cells convert tryptophan—an amino acid once widely sold over the counter as a sleep inducer—to melatonin. We now know melatonin declines with age and that it plays a major role in the sleep-wake cycle. Is the decline in the output of melatonin the reason older people have so many sleep problems?

Dr. D. Garfinkel and his colleagues at Tel Aviv University, Israel, reported in 1995 in *Lancet* the results of their studies on the effect of melatonin on the sleep quality of elderly people.[32] They gave twelve elderly subjects in their seventies, who were receiving various medications for chronic illnesses and who complained of insomnia, 2 mg of slow-release tablets of melatonin.

All the subjects, when tested, had lower peak excretion of melatonin during the night than normal in comparison to noninsomniac elderly. In a randomized, double-blind crossover study the subjects were treated for three weeks with 2 mg per night of controlled-release melatonin and for three weeks with placebo, with a week's washout period. Sleep quality was objectively monitored. Sleep efficiency was significantly greater after melatonin than after the placebo, and the wake time after sleep onset was significantly shorter. The time it took to fall asleep decreased, but not as significantly. Total sleep time was not affected. The only adverse effects reported were two cases of skin rash, one during melatonin and one during placebo treatment.

In other experiments, the researchers found that fast-release rather than slow-release melatonin only affected the onset of sleep rather than the total night's sleep.

The Israelis concluded that melatonin deficiency may have an important role in the high frequency of insomnia among elderly people. Controlled-release melatonin-replacement therapy effectively improves sleep quality in this population.

Richard Podell, M.D., clinical professor of medicine at the University of Medicine and Dentistry of New Jersey–Robert Wood Johnson Medical School, New Brunswick, and author of *Patient Power: How to Question Your Doctor* (Simon and Schus-

ter), says, "Melatonin is very interesting. It seems to work particularly well in older people with sleep problems. It is only anecdotal, but it seems to help 30 to 40 percent of the people. It also
works for jet lag. It seems to reduce sunburn effect and may be an
antioxidant and an antidepressant." He gives his patients half a
milligram to five milligrams, depending upon their needs.[33]

He says when he has prescribed melatonin for patients with
delayed-phase disorders—the night owl syndrome in which they
go to sleep late and wake up late—the hormone seems to reset
their sleep-wake cycle.

Dr. Podell notes melatonin is intimately related to serotonin
(a chemical messenger in the brain) and seems to raise it. If you
can increase serotonin, you may improve depression.

He says melatonin is contraindicated in winter depression because that is a high-melatonin state. It is also contraindicated in
manic-depressive disease and in any cancer of the immune system
and in autoimmune disease (see Glossary). On the other hand,
some studies show melatonin as an anticancer drug.

Dr. Alfred Lewy, an expert on biological clocks at Oregon
Health Sciences University, Portland, is worried about melatonin's potent effects on body "timing": "Before melatonin is
widely used, we need much more information on what to use it
for, how to use it, who will respond to it and who won't."

He says for example, if you want to avoid jet lag, melatonin
should be taken in the early morning if you are going west and in
the afternoon when going east; and since only varying amounts of
melatonin are needed to shift the body clock, Dr. Lewy also expressed concern about the dosages being sold, which he said may
be high enough to induce sleep at the wrong time in some people
who take it to counter jet lag.

"If you take it at the wrong time, you can create a body clock
disturbance—in effect, induce jet lag in yourself," Dr. Lewy advises.

In another study, researchers at Lyon Cedex, France, gave melatonin or a placebo to thirty-seven healthy volunteers on the day of a return jet flight and for three consecutive days. On day eight, self-ratings significantly discriminated between melatonin and placebo for treatment efficacy for morning fatigue and evening sleepiness.[34]

Some other studies show that you can reset your clock if you are crossing time zones by other means. For example:

- If staying in a new location more than two days, adopt local time for routines immediately upon arrival. If staying less than two days, maintain home schedule if possible.
- If staying more than two days, several days before departure try to gradually shift sleeping and eating routines to coincide with time at the destination.
- Before the flight, avoid overeating and alcohol.
- In flight, drink water and juices, not alcohol.
- If possible, break up long flights in one direction with lay-overs of at least a day.
- Allow plenty of time for sleep in the new location.
- After flying east, take walks outside in the morning to get used to the earlier appearance of light. Traveling eastward means shortening the day. This can be both difficult and stressful. After traveling west, take walks outside in the afternoon to acclimate to later waning of light. Traveling westward is easier for most people's biological clock adjustment. It means longer days, making it easier to deny oneself some sleep.

It usually takes three days in the new location to adapt all your body functions to the new time without the help of melatonin or the above efforts.

MELATONIN AND SEX

Melatonin's vaunted sexual benefits are "very muddled," says Dr. Lewy, who is a professor of psychiatry at Oregon Health Sciences University. Human mating isn't limited to fall or spring breeding cycles, as it is in those animals whose reproductive systems are most affected by melatonin, he advises, and an excess of it could theoretically dampen male libido and female fertility.

"I don't think people should take melatonin without consulting their doctor first," says Dr. Lewy. "Short-term experiments using melatonin as a sleep aid or jet-lag treatment haven't revealed any major toxicity yet. But hormones can take years to reveal their effects. It would be so nice to slip into melatonin like a pair of silk pajamas for the psyche. But nothing is that simple. For now, taking an unregulated sleep hormone demands open eyes and caveat emptor."

Fred W. Turek, director of the Center for Circadian Biology and Medicine at Northwestern University in Evanston, Illinois, who has researched melatonin for more than twenty years, is another who maintains there is scant or no evidence for these purported effects of melatonin as an anti-aging, antioxidant, or sex-enhancing compound. "Many of the claimed benefits of melatonin are based on a handful of small experiments or on individual testimonials, and the data are simply inconclusive," Turek wrote in the journal *Nature*.[35]

The "melatonin craze" resulted from some scientists' exaggerating the implications of their research to the media and to the general public, according to Turek. In the book *The Melatonin Miracle,* for instance, the authors "present many statements of fact about the health benefits of melatonin that, on closer inspection, often turn out to be merely hypotheses with little supportive data," he said.

Dr. Turek has coauthored a "white paper" with Dr. Charles

Czeisler of Brigham and Women's Hospital in Boston. The paper was commissioned by the National Sleep Foundation. It asserts that the use of melatonin "cannot be justified for any sleep disorder at this time, since neither the therapeutic nor potential toxic effects of prolonged use have been documented." Of particular concern, the researchers note, is that melatonin has been shown to have a "profound effect on the reproductive systems" of many animals.

The paper, "Possible Role for Melatonin in the Treatment of Insomnia and Jet Lag," summarizes nearly fifteen years of research and references forty studies. It concludes, "Preliminary data in humans indicate that melatonin may have sleep-inducing properties and may induce phase shifts in human rhythms," seeming to make the hormone "an attractive candidate for treating sleep disorders related to inappropriate circadian timing."

The report notes, however, that many clinical studies of melatonin suffer from methodological flaws such as having subjects rate the length and quality of their own sleep.

Before melatonin can legitimately be recommended as a sleep aid, "carefully controlled clinical trials that focus on the possible beneficial effects of melatonin on specific sleep disorders are urgently needed," the authors conclude.

A two-day NIH workshop held August 12–13, 1996, in Bethesda, Maryland, issued similar precautions about unregulated use of the hormone. At the workshop, Dr. Daniel Kripke of the University of California at San Diego presented data on forty-two subjects between the ages of sixty and seventy-nine who had been diagnosed with insomnia. After two years, Dr. Kripke said, the trial shows no correlation between levels of self-produced melatonin and minutes of sleep and suggests that a link between low melatonin levels and increased insomnia is "doubtful."

Dr. Kripke said further analysis of his data is expected to determine the relationship, if any, between melatonin levels and onset of sleepiness and will take about five years.

His data showed that ten to twelve urine samples taken during each of two twenty-four-hour collection periods showed that melatonin levels did not peak at night in all subjects, suggesting that melatonin may not, in fact, be a "night hormone" for elderly populations.

This preliminary data, combined with information from animal and clinical studies about possible gonadal atrophy and suppression of luteinizing hormones related to melatonin use, suggests that the hormone should not yet be recommended for long-term use, Dr. Kripke stated.

There were some positive findings, however, at the NIH melatonin workshop. Dr. Robert Sack, Oregon Health Sciences University, presented research indicating that melatonin "may be helpful" to night workers in shifting to an inverted schedule of work and sleep.

The double-blind trial enrolled twenty-seven hospital personnel who worked on a schedule requiring seven consecutive ten-hour night shifts alternating with one week off. The workers received either 5-mg gelatin capsules of melatonin or placebo capsules on a regimented schedule to test melatonin's effect on their ability to adjust their circadian rhythms to match their changing schedules.

Melatonin seemed to aid "resetting" of sleep patterns in about half of the sixteen subjects who otherwise had no or incomplete shifts in their sleep-wake patterns.

Richard J. Wurtman, M.D., a professor of neuroscience and director of the clinical research center at the Massachusetts Institute of Technology in Boston, and one of the prime melatonin researchers, also warns that overuse of melatonin may cause problems: "Melatonin probably can help some people with insomnia or jet lag, but to suggest that a woman with breast cancer or someone with HIV could help their conditions by taking melatonin is dangerously wicked."

Dr. Wurtman says, "There is not a shred of evidence that people with cancer or HIV respond" to supplemental melatonin.

Another concern of Dr. Wurtman's is the way melatonin is being sold: "The dose of the hormone that has been shown to raise nighttime blood levels of melatonin to those of people with normal sleep patterns is 0.3 milligram. But melatonin is often sold at doses of up to 3 milligrams, which is ten times the amount needed for a normal night's sleep, and there may be side effects from such a high dose."[36]

The problem, according to MIT's Dr. Wurtman is that the melatonin sold in health-food stores is unregulated. "There's a reason we have a Food and Drug Administration," Dr.Wurtman stressed in an interview with *Neurology Reviews,* and again at a meeting at the National Institutes of Health, Bethesda, Maryland, August 12, 1996. In tests at his laboratory, impurities were found in some of the melatonin samples obtained at health-food stores. "We don't want to reexperience the tryptophan tragedy," in which serious illness and deaths were linked with impurities in an unregulated product, said Dr. Wurtman.[37]

At 3-mg doses, melatonin induces a sleep hangover, Dr. Wurtman said, adding that "I still don't know whether or not people taking it at that dose will be fit to drive twenty-four hours later." Taking too much could induce round-the-clock drowsiness, hypothermia, a loss of infection-fighting power, and a rise in the hormone prolactin. "If you're a man, this decreases your sex drive," he says. If you're a woman with a slow-growing breast cancer that is prolactin-sensitive, he fears its growth could accelerate.

But there's more to the controversy. As Dr. Wurtman readily admits, his interest in melatonin is financial as well as educational. As a result of his research, MIT has applied for a patent for melatonin's use in sleep disorders and has licensed the patent application rights to Interneuron Pharmaceuticals, Inc., a small company in Lexington, Massachusetts. Dr. Wurtman cofounded Interneuron in 1988 and is a major stockholder and chairman of its scientific advisory board. As a result of this connection, a story in the *Wall Street Journal* reported that Dr. Wurtman "is drawing charges of blurring the boundaries between research and commerce in his work on melatonin."[38]

"I absolutely am!" Dr. Wurtman told *Neurology Reviews*. "But as a matter of national policy, I think we want that blurring to take place. The alternative is that we never have anything of therapeutic value come out of our universities."

Dr. Wurtman explained, "Prior to the mid-1970s, it was rare for universities to obtain patents on their research. As a result, they had a difficult time finding pharmaceutical sponsors to conduct the expensive, large-scale clinical trials on their laboratory discoveries that would ultimately yield marketable therapeutics. The trend toward obtaining patents, however, only partially solved the problem. For the most part, pharmaceutical companies still prefer to promote their own research rather than obtain a license to someone else's patent.

"Nevertheless, the universities don't have the money necessary for large-scale trials," Dr. Wurtman continued. When presented with an opportunity to help found a company that would invest in trials involving some of MIT's patents, Dr. Wurtman agreed.

His research-commerce relationship has limits. As a stockholder in Interneuron, Dr. Wurtman is prevented by MIT from accepting financial support from Interneuron for his research. And MIT is under no obligation to license his patents to Interneuron. He noted that often, however, there are no other bidders.

Dr. Robert Sack, a professor of psychiatry at Oregon Health Sciences University in Portland, has found that melatonin can help elderly insomniacs as well as night-shift workers who need to sleep during the day. The benefits of melatonin for jet lag also have been fairly well established, he said.

But beyond these uses, there is no evidence of any other therapeutic effect from melatonin, Sack says, adding, "The claims for living to be 130 years old are kind of a long shot."[39]

Dr. Sack pointed out at the National Institutes of Health meeting in 1996 that "we are going at it backwards....People are taking it [melatonin], and we are trying to figure out what it does."[40]

Sack said the over-the-counter use of melatonin is "sort of an uncontrolled experiment. We are nervous about that."

Hormones have a wide range of actions and interactions throughout the body. Aside from inducing sleep, melatonin also lowers fertility (some consider it a potential contraceptive). It may further affect immune reactions in ways not fully understood. So while some researchers are testing it as a companion to chemotherapy for certain cancers, its immunologic ripple effects could potentially promote other tumors.

Melatonin has been banned in Britain and France, and some countries regulate it as a drug. Italy and Denmark cracked down on companies touting its purported medical benefits.

Consider the source. Some melatonin products are extracted from cow pineal glands. With concern mounting over the spread of brain-destroying "mad cow" disease from cattle to humans, it might be wise to avoid unregulated products of bovine brain. Synthetic forms of the product lack this risk.

The National Institute on Aging's Dr. Monjan advises, "Buyer beware. In preliminary studies with young and old persons, melatonin seems to have some positive results, but there are a number of factors that have to be established":

- What is the proper dose?
- What are the types of conditions resulting in sleep distur-bances that can be helped by melatonin?
- What are the long-term effects?[41]

Dr. Monjan says that short term there don't seem to be ad-verse effects in healthy individuals, but what is yet to be deter-mined is melatonin's interactions with other health conditions such as diabetes, autoimmune disease, pregnancy, and depression.

SLEEP AND DHEA

DHEA (dehydroepiandrosterone) is another controversial hor-mone that is said to have many benefits. Derived from the adrenal gland, its administration increases rapid eye movement sleep and EEG power in the sigma frequency range during REM sleep.[42] It exhibits various behavioral effects in mammals, at least one of which is enhancement of memory, which appears to be mediated by an interaction with the gamma-aminobutyric acid (GABA) re-ceptor complex. GABA is found in high concentrations in the brain and functions as an inhibitory chemical messenger.

A dose of five hundred milligrams of DHEA was given to ten healthy young men to determine its effects on sleep stages, with a sleep-stage-specific EEG used to monitor brain waves. DHEA ad-ministration induced a significant increase in rapid eye movement (REM) sleep during the first two hours of sleep, whereas all other sleep variables remained unchanged compared with the placebo condition. Because REM sleep has been implicated in memory storage, its augmentation in the present study suggests the poten-tial clinical usefulness of DHEA in age-related dementia.

In another experiment, male cadets at a Norwegian military facility were tested during five days of continuous heavy physical activities with little or no food and sleep. Blood levels of DHEA, testosterone, and thyroid-stimulating hormones were examined. The normal twenty-four-hour circadian rhythm nearly disappeared. Mental performance, of course, decreased. The circadian rhythms of the thyroid and testosterone hormones were almost normalized after four or five days, but the adrenal hormones were not. This led the Norwegian researchers to conclude that the "stress" hormones of the adrenal gland take longer to recover their normal circadian rhythm.[43]

The Norwegian experiment was with young men at the top of their physical fitness. What happens when lack of sleep and proper nutrition occurs in more vulnerable old people?

A good night's sleep keeps the brain in good working order. The loss of cognitive power seems in some way related to an inability to maintain a restful sleep. Insomnia and disturbed sleep patterns are not found in all older people. Therefore, it may well be that poor sleep is abnormal, if somewhat common, as we age. Furthermore, much insomnia and restless sleep may be due to psychological problems rather than physiologic ones. Many older people have nothing to do during the day. They catnap and have no set routine. Therefore, they may awaken at night because they had sufficient sleep during the day.

It may be that a deficiency in melatonin and/or DHEA as we age causes some of us sleep problems. Human sleep is regulated by a concerted action of various chemicals acting on sleep-generating nerves in the brain whose night activity is not fully understood. During sleep, however, it is known that hormones are very active.[44] Hormones can also keep us from sleeping. We don't need scientists to tell us that when we are under stress, we often suffer from insomnia. Now, Alexandros Vgontzas, M.D., and his colleagues at Penn State's Milton S. Hershey Medical Center found that people with chronic insomnia had higher levels of cortisol, a hormone secreted when the body is under stress. In the study, Dr. Vgontzas and his team followed nine insomniacs who were not taking any medication and who did not have any major mental illness. The researchers found that the chronic insomniacs had higher levels of stress hormones but now wonder whether it's the stress that keeps people awake or the insomnia that is the source of the stress.[45]

The study also measured the effect of chronic insomnia on growth hormone. In all subjects, the levels of growth hormone were extremely low, providing further evidence that the immune system is chronically stressed. An active stress system is known to reduce growth hormone secretion.

As many university researchers and government scientists point out, however, hormones are powerful chemicals that can do wonderful things if properly used, but because of their capabilities, they can pose dangers if not used appropriately—even though they may easily be purchased over the counter.

7. TESTOSTERONE—REPLACEMENT THERAPY AND VIRILITY

Avoiding Age-Associated Dysfunctions

Is testosterone an "anti-aging" hormone for men? Will TRT (testosterone replacement therapy) soon be as common as ERT (estrogen replacement therapy)? The idea of giving supplemental testosterone to combat signs of male aging such as flagging virility and loss of muscle strength is certainly not new.

In 1848, a German professor, Arnold Berthold, transplanted healthy poultry testicles to the chests of two desexed roosters, and the capons began again to chase "chicks" around the coop.

A generation later, Charles Edouard Brown-Sequard, a highly respected professor of experimental medicine at the Sorbonne in Paris, shocked his colleagues by performing a similar experiment —on himself.

In 1869, he suggested that the injection of semen into the blood of old men might stimulate their mental and physical powers. He was content, at that time, merely to voice the suggestion to his close colleagues. As he grew older, however, the idea of rejuvenation became more and more intriguing to him. In 1875, he attempted a series of testicular grafts on guinea pigs. Then, one languid June night, at age seventy-two, he made a startling announcement before his colleagues at the French Academy of Medicine. He claimed he had rejuvenated himself with injections of a saline extract of dogs' testicles.

"Everything I have not been able to do for several years on account of my advanced age," he asserted, "I am, today, able to perform most admirably." He continued, "Behold the results. Miracle of miracles, and wonders of wonders. After only a few injections I can work for hours. I stand up in the laboratory instead of sitting down. And when I get home, I eat a hearty supper and return once more to my work."

His colleagues were skeptical, but Brown-Sequard continued his experiments, and when he reported the same results a few weeks later, they burst into applause. The Paris papers heralded his findings on their front pages, and other erudite groups, as well as the worldwide press, became interested.

When Brown-Sequard's results could not be reproduced, the scientific community labeled the experiments quackery and Charles Brown-Sequard a crazy old man. Actually, Brown-Sequard may have been one hundred years ahead of his time. The incident, however, set back the study of endocrinology for years because young scientists were reluctant to take up the study of glands lest they be tainted by Brown-Sequard's supposed folly.

Brown-Sequard was certainly not the first to associate testicles with virility. Adult males have focused on their testicles since ancient times. History contains references to experiments with bull testicles to restore human male potency as far back as 1500 B.C. In fact, enemy testicles were often brought back by soldiers as the trophies of war, and our language contains words such as *testify, testy,* and *testimonial*, which shows how males once swore on their testicles before they swore on the Bible.

The testicles, those most important male sex glands, are contained in the scrotal sac between the legs. They produce testosterone. This hormone has two major effects: **androgenic,** to stimulate the appearance of secondary sexual characteristics at puberty, such as the growth of body hair, deepening of the voice, an increase in the size of the genitals, and the production of sperm; **anabolic,** to increase muscle bulk, accelerate rate of growth.

WILL TESTOSTERONE AND OTHER MALE HORMONES RESTORE YOUTHFUL FUNCTIONING?

As in women—but not as dramatically—the male body's ability to use male hormones declines with the passing years. As a result, some changes in human male sexual function are almost universally associated with aging. They are:

- **A longer period of time needed to reach an erection.**
  Some interesting work has been done to actually measure the change. Two researchers at the University of Southern California showed the same erotic movie to two groups of men and measured their responses. The men who were between nineteen and thirty years of age developed erections almost six times faster than the men between forty-eight and sixty-five years old.
- **An erection that may be slightly less firm than when a man was younger.**
- **It is easier to delay orgasm and ejaculation.** This can be a plus for a female lover who may take longer to arouse.
- **Ejaculation is less forceful.** For some men, the ejaculation is also slightly less pleasurable.
- **Less fluid is ejaculated.**
- **After orgasm, erection is lost more quickly.**
- **There's a longer period of "down time" between erections.**

A man will usually experience these changes over a period of many years, generally beginning in his thirties. Typically, they come on gradually and sometimes are so subtle they won't be noticed for a long time. Many of these changes will be insignificant; some will be welcome; some will require adjustment.

In addition, muscle size and strength decreases, body fat increases and hair thins. The most common type of hair loss is pattern baldness, a hereditary trait that is expressed more often in males than in females because it depends on the influence of male hormones. Pattern baldness in males extends until only a sparse growth of hair remains on the back and sides of the head. In women, the baldness usually extends until only a sparse growth remains on the crown.

THE SUCCESSFUL SEARCH FOR THE MALE ESSENCE

Can hormone supplementation restore youthful function and appearance to an aging male body? Was poor old Brown-Sequard really on the right track but with the wrong species?

It was bull testicles that led to the ultimately successful search for the "male essence." In 1926, University of Chicago professor of physiologic chemistry, Fred C. Koch, and his student-assistant, Lemuel McGee, ground up bulls' testicles and prepared one extract after another. When they assayed them by the capon-comb test, some compounds displayed a little more male activity than others. But none showed enough activity to be labeled even "promising."

After two years, the small grant under which Koch and McGee had worked ran out and was not renewed. Undaunted, however, Fred Koch spent his own salary to purchase more bulls' testicles and gallons of solvents. In 1929, he and Dr. T. F. Gallagher finally developed a many-staged extraction process that yielded a mixture much more active than any Koch had ever before been able to prepare. Whereas it had taken weeks for his old extracts to evoke even a little growth in a capon's withered comb, one hundredth of a milligram of this new substance produced an upstanding red comb in just five days.

Unlike Brown-Sequard's startling announcement before the French Academy, Fred Koch wrote a dry and factual report. He ended it with a cautionary declaration. "The product is as yet grossly impure....It should not be given a chemical name."

Koch's report was not buried and forgotten as Professor Berthold's capon experiments had been. Other researchers became interested, among them a German biochemist, Adolf Friedrich Johann Butenandt, who had extracted the female hormones, estrone in 1929 and progesterone in 1934. Using urine rather than testicles, Butenandt managed to isolate a few grains of crystalline male hormone in 1931. Because it stimulated cock comb growth and because it was a steroid, he coined a Greek name for it, *androsterone*. While androsterone was biologically active, it was soon found to be not the male hormone itself but a metabolically changed or degraded form of it.

By 1935, a team working under the Dutch pharmacologist Dr. Ernest Laqueur and using an improved variant of Koch's earlier method, succeeded in extracting the true male hormone, *testosterone*, from bulls' testicles.

Just one year later, a Croatian-born Swiss organic chemist, Leopold Ruzicka, synthesized androsterone and testosterone in his laboratory. His patent for the preparation of testosterone from cholesterol earned him a fortune.[1]

He and Adolph Butenandt shared the 1939 Nobel Prize for chemistry for their work on isolating and synthesizing male hormones.

THE GOOD AND BAD OF MALE HORMONES

Until recently, most modern scientists believed that testosterone, the major male hormone, might be more destructive to the male than constructive. In fact, some theorized that women live so much longer than men because they have less of it.

A long-term study of institutionalized mentally retarded males was published in 1970, involving 735 uncastrated males and 297 eunuchs. Each eunuch was closely matched with one or more intact males for such characteristics as year of birth and length of hospitalization.[2] Because of their genetic retardation, the subjects had only a vague idea of the effects of castration, which reduced any possible adverse psychological effects of the operation.

The average life span for the intact males was 55.7 years, and for the eunuchs, 69.3. The younger the males were castrated, the longer they lived. However, for most normal males, obviously, when it comes to a choice between virility and a longer life, most would certainly choose virility.

The study also indicated that the castrated are less susceptible to infections. This is believed to be due to the antibody-lowering effect of testosterone reported by some researchers. Antibodies are the body's disease fighters.

Do more virile men—those with high levels of testosterone— die younger? Statistics show that ambitious, aggressive men are more prone to heart disease than others. Studies performed under grants from the National Institutes of Health show that the higher the level of testosterone, the more aggressive the man.[3]

This observation would not surprise farmers. They know how the fierce bull after castration becomes docile, and how the rooster, caponized to make his meat more tender, becomes far less "cocky." Those who have feline pets are probably aware that if you want a tomcat to stop howling, marking, and roaming, removing his testicles can keep him sleeping peacefully at home. While some wives might wish to keep their husbands sleeping peacefully at home, "alteration" is not a good option. In fact, both men and women have an interest in keeping up normal levels of male hormone for both mental and physical well-being in maturity. As with any active chemical substance, however, there are benefits and potentially unwanted side effects.

SEX HORMONES ARE IN THE HEAD AS WELL AS THE TESTICLES

We all know that what we think can affect us sexually, but what goes on physically inside a man's brain can also have an enormous impact on his erections—specifically, what goes on inside his pituitary gland.

Just a little bigger than a peanut without its shell, located in a recess within the skull behind the nose, the pituitary gland produces a hormone (luteinizing hormone) that tells the testicles to produce yet another hormone—testosterone—which is necessary for potency.

Gonadotropins are hormones that influence the development and functioning of the ovaries and testes. The main source of follicle-stimulating hormone (FSH) and luteinizing hormone in both men and women is the anterior portion of the pituitary.[4] A great deal of research is in progress to determine the effects of the gonadotropins in aging and whether supplementation may be beneficial. This work, however, is far behind the research in progress with the major male hormones, testosterone and androgen.

What happens to male hormones in the very old? Researchers at the University of Bologna in Italy wanted to find out, so they studied 150 healthy males ranging in age from 27 to 103 years.[5] All were self-sufficient, nonhospitalized, clean-living guys.

As other researchers have found, the Italian investigators, led by Dr. G. Ravaglia, reported that free testosterone begins to decrease in about the fourth decade. They discovered, however, the first significant decrease in total testosterone was found only in men over ninety. The oldest group also had higher levels of gonadotropins, sex hormone stimulators from the brain and pituitary. The researchers reasoned that this was a simple consequence of the marked deficit in testicular hormone production.

Dr. Ravaglia and his colleagues did not state in their paper whether the old, old men were sexually active, but they did express admiration: "The excellent psychophysical conditions of the old-old people which we studied make these subjects practically a group on their own, for whom the processes of senescence seem to have occurred much more favorably with respect to the majority of the elderly population. In spite of this, the data show how, precisely in this group apparently immune to the effects of aging, the changes in their male hormone levels were significantly evident."

MALE HORMONE SUPPLEMENTATION

Would the healthy, independent-living Italian men over ninety with low levels of male hormones benefit from supplementation? Their longevity is obviously not dependent on it. The researchers at the University of Bologna point out that "the physiology of aging in very old people is still poorly understood and that a wide variety of age-related factors confuse the interpretation of existing data, especially in regards to the modifications of the endocrine system."[6]

New research is studying testosterone as an anti-aging hormone. A number of synthetically produced derivatives of testosterone produce varying degrees of the androgenic and anabolic effects mentioned above. Taken in low doses as part of replacement therapy when natural production is low, male sex hormones act in the same way as the natural hormones. Those having a mainly anabolic effect are known as *anabolic steroids* and are sold under names such as Nandrolone and Oxandrolone. Testosterone, which is primarily *androgenic,* is sold in a number of forms—

pills, patches, and injections—under such names as Testoderm Scrotal Patch, Testogect-LA, and Testred Cypionate.

THE ANABOLIC STEROIDS

Anabolic steroids derived from testosterone came to public notice following World War II, when they were used to restore body weight in concentration camp survivors. The drugs are sometimes given today to "build up"—to stimulate growth, weight gain, strength, and appetite. Physicians occasionally prescribe anabolic steroids and a high-protein diet to promote recovery after a severe illness, injury, surgery, continuing infection, or when, for unknown reasons, patients fail to gain or maintain normal weight. Anabolic steroids have also been used in the treatment of the bone-wasting disorder osteoporosis, breast cancer, and hereditary angioedema, which causes swelling of the face, arms, legs, and throat. Anabolics may also help to increase the production of blood cells in some forms of anemia.

In the early 1950s the drugs were widely employed by athletes in the hope of enhancing performance. In conjunction with an intensive exercise training program and high-protein diet, these drugs can indeed increase muscle bulk, which may improve performance in certain sports. They speed up the recovery of muscles after a session of intense exercise. This enables the athlete to go through a more demanding daily exercise program, resulting in a significant improvement in muscle power. Anabolic steroids can have serious side effects, however, and young athletes abusing them are at risk for premature closure of the growth plates of the long bones. All athletes misusing anabolics are in danger of causing sterility, liver damage, cancer, and even death. Female athletes may also develop male-pattern baldness and facial hair. These drugs can, in addition, produce high levels of aggression in both sexes.

Anabolic steroids drew world attention in 1988 when Canadian sprinter Ben Johnson was stripped of his Olympic gold medal after tests indicated steroid use. Less widely publicized was the epidemic steroid abuse among high school and college athletes in many sports in the United States.

On February 27, 1991, anabolic steroids became controlled drugs requiring prescriptions and record keeping. The U.S. Olympic Committee and the National Collegiate Athletic Association have also banned the use of male hormones by athletes to build muscle strength.

Controlled use of anabolic steroids, of course, does have medicinal benefits in persons who are deficient in the male hormone or who have health conditions that may respond to therapeutic dosages, as pointed out before.

Anabolic steroids may be widely abused, but can testosterone be employed to increase strength in aging men who are not deficient in the hormone? Researchers from the Charles Drew University of Medicine and Science, Los Angeles, and Exercise Science Laboratory, El Camino College, in Torrance, California, sought to determine that.[7] They randomly assigned forty-three normal men to one of four groups:

- Placebo with no exercise
- Testosterone with no exercise
- Placebo plus exercise
- Testosterone plus exercise[8]

The men received injections of 600 mg of testosterone or placebo weekly for ten weeks. The participants in the exercise groups performed standardized weight-lifting exercises three times weekly. Before and after the treatment period, fat-free mass was determined by underwater weighing, muscle size was measured by magnetic resonance imaging, and the strength of the arms and legs were assessed by bench-press and squatting exercises, respectively.

Among the subjects in the no-exercise groups, those given testosterone had greater increases than those given a placebo in muscle size in their arms and greater increases in strength in the bench-press and the squatting exercises. The men assigned to testosterone and exercise had greater increases in fat-free mass and muscle size, and greater increases in muscle strength, than men in any of the other groups. Neither mood nor behavior was altered in any group.

The California researchers concluded that increasing testosterone above normal levels, especially when combined with strength training, increases fat-free mass and muscle size and strength in normal men. The lead researcher, Shalender Bhasin, M.D., and colleagues warned, however, their results "in no way justify the use of anabolic-androgenic steroids in sports, because with extended use, such drugs have potentially serious adverse effects on the cardiovascular system, prostate, lipid metabolism, and insulin sensitivity. Moreover, the use of any performance-enhancing agent in sports raises serious ethical issues."[9]

They said their findings do, however, raise the possibility that short-term administration of androgens may have beneficial effects in immobilized patients, during space travel, and in patients with cancer-related loss of appetite, disease caused by AIDS, or other chronic wasting disorders including those associated with very old age.

Declining testosterone in HIV-positive men may be an early signal for the dangerous weight loss that occurs when AIDS develops, according to a Johns Hopkins study.[10] "A drop in testosterone may be an early way to identify patients at risk for losing too much weight," says Adrian S. Dobs, M.D., lead author and associate professor of medicine. "Helping them prevent or slow weight loss may become an important new treatment for AIDS."

Results of the study, funded by the National Institutes of Health, were presented June 12, 1996, at the International Congress of Endocrinology's annual meeting in San Francisco. In a related study, Hopkins researchers recently found that HIV-positive men who lose too much weight before developing AIDS are at risk for earlier death than those who maintain their weight. Two other ongoing Hopkins studies are investigating whether testosterone injections and testosterone skin patches help HIV-positive men regain lean body weight, possibly increasing life span and improving their quality of life. If the studies show the hormone is effective, researchers plan to test whether testosterone given before weight loss prevents wasting.

Researchers measured testosterone in twenty-six men infected with the human immunodeficiency virus (HIV) to determine if hormone changes preceded or were linked to wasting (the loss of enough weight to cause illness) or if the weight loss caused the decline in hormones. Half the men had lost more than 10 percent of their original weight without diarrhea and opportunistic infections, while the other half had gained weight.

Researchers found six months later that testosterone levels had declined significantly in all thirteen men who lost at least 10 percent of their weight, while testosterone levels stayed the same in thirteen men who gained or maintained their weight. The men losing weight also lost white blood cells, which help fight infection. In AIDS, the virus damages certain white blood cells, called T cells, crippling the body's ability to defeat infections.

Increased risk of death due to wasting is caused in part by an increase in the body's metabolic rate, the speed with which the body burns up food. Severe diarrhea and infections that strike AIDS patients whose immune systems are crippled can overwhelm the person's ability to maintain their weight, say researchers. Aging also weakens the immune system.

Hair Today and Wrinkles Tomorrow

Strong muscles and a lean body may be symbols of youthful vigor for men, but what about other common manifestations of the passing years—a bald head and wrinkled skin?

Jean L. Bolognia, M.D., of the Department of Dermatology at Yale Medical School, wrote in a 1995 paper published by the *American Journal of Medicine:* "Some of the skin changes that have been categorized as secondary to chronologic aging, such as decreased sebaceous [oil] gland activity and decreased hair growth, may actually represent a decline in the concentration of tissue androgens with increasing age."[11]

Dr. Bolognia urged that while the influence of androgens on age-related changes in the skin and hair remains speculative, there is "obvious need for studies in this area."

Testosterone Supplementation

What about testosterone as an anti-aging hormone? Just like old professor Brown-Sequard, many of today's men would "go to the dogs" to restore their youthful sexual vigor if that were necessary.

Behind the penis are the *testicles,* two ball-shaped endocrine glands that are vital to erection and the production of testosterone. In the womb, a male fetus's testicles actually change location. They form near the kidneys but during the last three months of pregnancy descend into the bag that holds them, the scrotum. The testicles are vulnerable and quite sensitive to even minor injuries such as a fall off a bike or an awkward landing from a height. The production of male hormones in the testicles is more resistant to environmental hazards. Yet, just how testosterone influences erection is still something of a mystery. Some men with erection problems have low testosterone levels, and they can successfully be treated with supplemental hormone. However, some men with low levels of the hormones have no problems getting and maintaining erections.[12]

Testosterone is essential to sexual desire. With just a bare minimum of it, a man's sexual desire is greatly reduced or nonexistent, and he has a decreased volume of ejaculate and a general malaise.

Testosterone levels fall naturally as a man ages, but the decline is gradual and the impact is not as dramatic as the sudden loss of estrogen in women. More than 60 percent of men by age sixty-five have low levels of male hormone.[13] Blood levels of testosterone below the lower normal limit occur, however, only in a minority of elderly men: 7 percent in those forty to sixty, 20 percent in those sixty to eighty, and 35 percent in those over eighty.[14] The factors influencing testosterone levels in elderly men are multiple, according to researchers, and include heredity, obesity, stress, depression, smoking, drugs, diet, and hygiene.[15]

St. Louis University Medical School's Fran Kaiser, M.D., associate director of geriatric medicine, has reported that giving men an injectable form of testosterone for three months increases their muscle strength and sex drive and counters anemia.[16]

She and her colleagues studied a group of twelve males over age seventy. The six men given regular injections of testosterone over a three-month period not only experienced a gain in weight and muscle strength, but their cholesterol levels dropped and their bones became stronger as well. Earlier studies have indicated that men with low levels of testosterone are six times as likely to break a hip when they fall than those with normal testosterone levels.

British researchers at the Bone Clinic, Freeman Hospital, Newcastle upon Tyne, described the case of a seventy-four-year-old man with a four-month history of lower-back pain and progressive loss of height of three inches. Endocrine assessment showed he had slightly lower serum testosterone—he was not offered testosterone replacement by his regular physician "as it was felt it would be of little value in a man of his age."[17]

The Bone Clinic doctors started the man on fortnightly intramuscular injections of 250 mg of testosterone. That was in 1989. The physicians reported in a *Lancet* article that the man "noted an improvement in back pain and a sense of well-being on treatment....Although his increased libido caused some marital problems."

The doctors then lowered his dose of testosterone, his wife was happy, and X rays showed an increase in bone density over the next four years. The man continues happy on testosterone treatment at age eighty-one.

"But not every man needs supplemental testosterone since not everyone has low levels of male hormone," Dr. Kaiser cautions. "Most physicians just consider the total level of testosterone in the blood, and that is not an accurate indication of whether a deficiency exists. The significant factor is bioavailability—what the body actually can use."

Dr. Kaiser says it "absolutely scares me when I see television shows promoting a new testosterone patch as a 'passion patch.'"[18] She says a lot of people are going to get sucked in and will be given testosterone when they don't need it.

"One of the first questions we ask men who want to enter the testosterone replacement therapy is 'How tall were you?'" Dr. Kaiser says. "Most of the men have lost height because they have osteoporosis, and testosterone is beneficial to men's bones in the same way that estrogen is to women's."

She says the men who are in the program want to stay in it because it makes them feel better and increases their strength and sex drive.

"One sixty-two-year-old professional who had a low testosterone level was down in the dumps but not clinically depressed, because we screen out those who are," she continues, and he had low self-esteem, lack of strength upon exercising, and a low sex drive. "We put him on testosterone and all his symptoms reversed, and his wife was even happier as a side benefit. But the man had one of the potential side effects, polycythemia—an overproduction of red blood cells. He refused to stop the testosterone, so he had to undergo the treatment for polycythemia, which is taking a unit of blood off periodically.

"We had another man with the same side effect who chose to drop out, but in four months he was back, asking to be readmitted."

She said that most men by age fifty have a decline in testosterone, but that does not mean they need supplementation. The St. Louis program accepts only those who have significantly low bioavailable testosterone.

The National Institute on Aging is sponsoring studies at the University of Pennsylvania and at Emory University in Atlanta on testosterone replacement in men sixty-five and over. The researchers are measuring changes in energy level, bone density, mental function, muscle mass, strength, and body fat, all of which may be affected by supplemental testosterone.

Dr. Kaiser said the biggest concern is that boosting testosterone levels in some men can also boost their risk for strokes by increasing red blood cell counts, and if someone has prostate cancer, it could grow faster. A study by researchers at the University of South Carolina found that testosterone regulates thromboxane A2, a substance that causes vasoconstriction and blood clotting that has been implicated in heart and blood-vessel disease.[19] On the other hand, researchers from the Department of Family and Preventive Medicine, University of California, found that testosterone levels in the high normal range appear to be conducive to "optimal cardiovascular health for adult men."[20]

Dr. Kaiser says testosterone should not be taken orally because that form may cause liver damage. She and her colleagues prescribe the hormone by injection or by a skin patch.

How Do You Know You Have Low Testosterone?

Your body has warning signs: low energy, listlessness, a lack of sex drive, and erection problems. But the only sure way to know if testosterone is lacking is to get a blood test. However, because a man's testosterone level is not constant, but rises in spurts, pooling of several samples to get an accurate measure may be necessary.

The effect of hormones on erections is still something of a mystery. Some men with low testosterone experience dramatic improvement when they get extra amounts to bring them up to normal. What's confusing is that not all men with low testosterone suffer from the effects of it, as pointed out before. Some are able to get normal erections without difficulty. Dr. Kaiser says, "A man with normal levels of testosterone will not get better erections if he takes unneeded supplements of the hormone, but his desire may increase—and he may endanger his health. The fact that we can't say absolutely what is normal for any particular man makes the treatment of men with borderline low testosterone somewhat of a judgment call."

Dr. Kaiser advises testosterone levels should be measured carefully: "Free testosterone levels are worthless. The levels of bioavailable testosterone that the body can use is what should be measured. A man should never, ever, be put on testosterone without measuring the levels of hormone, making sure his levels are low. Why give some normal men testosterone? Many men after the age of sixty years have hormone levels that go down, but men don't have menstrual periods that stop, so there is no visible marker. For those with low testosterone level, replacement, short term, can have benefits. It may have a major impact on sex drive and on upper-arm strength, and energy level does seem to pick up. But we need long-term studies."[21]

In adult men, the effects of testosterone supplements on physical appearance and libido may begin to be felt within a few weeks.[22]

Women and Testosterone

Women's ovaries and adrenal glands provide a modest amount of testosterone. Production rates in normal women average 0.2 mg a day with 24 percent secreted by the ovaries, 25 percent by the adrenals, and 50 percent arising from the peripheral metabolism of prehormones such as DHEA.[23] But what happens when the ovaries begin to shut down? The exact function of testosterone in the female body is not known. Researchers at Beth Israel Medical Center, New York, measured testosterone in thirty-three healthy, nonobese women between twenty-one and fifty-one years of age over a twenty-four-hour period. From that study, they calculate that testosterone concentration in a woman of forty years is about half that of a woman of twenty-one.[24]

Some scientific reports and even a popular book have purported that testosterone supplementation boosts women's response to estrogen replacement therapy and also makes them more interested in sex.[25] Australian researchers at Prince Henry's Institute of Medical Research gave thirty-four postmenopausal women either estrogen implants of 50 mg alone or with 50 mg of testosterone. The implants were administered every three months for two years. Cyclical oral progestins were taken by women who still had an intact uterus. Of the thirty-two women who completed the study, bone and spine density increased significantly in both treatment groups. At all sites the bone density increased more rapidly in the testosterone-treated group. Sexual parameters improved significantly in both groups. The addition of testosterone, however, the Australians reported, resulted in a significantly greater improvement in satisfaction, pleasure, and orgasm. Total cholesterol in both groups fell, as did total body fat. They concluded that the benefits of estrogen on blood fats was maintained in women treated with testosterone and that the testosterone implants were of benefit for diminished libido in postmenopausal women.

Dr. Kaiser, however, is against testosterone's use in women: "It is given to increase low sex drive. If you raise the level of testosterone in women, you may change her risk of heart and blood-vessel disease and high blood pressure. There are other side effects, such as deepening of the voice, acne, and increased hair growth."[26]

High doses may also produce enlargement of the clitoris and changes in libido. Researchers have also found that while increased levels of testosterone in men are associated with decreased blood sugar concentrations, in "striking contrast" women have high blood sugar and insulin resistance with increased levels of male hormones.[27]

British researchers maintain that giving small doses of testosterone avoids such side effects. The Londoners purported in a review article published in the *American Journal of Medicine,* "Women who are androgen depleted develop physical and behavioral symptoms referred to as *female androgen deficiency syndrome.*"[28] To a lesser degree, women who undergo an oophorectomy (removal of the ovaries) are deprived of endogenous ovarian androgens and have consistently been shown to have impairment of sexual functioning, loss of energy, depression, and headaches. The researchers, who are in the department of obstetrics and gynecology at Chelsea and Westminster Hospital, maintain testosterone seems to act synergistically with estrogen in the treatment of these symptoms.

The combination of estrogen and testosterone has been shown to have a beneficial effect on the skeleton, although not significantly better than estrogen therapy alone.

The Londoners conclude that androgen replacement therapy is a neglected area of medical practice and that further research is needed to identify all women who will benefit from it since studies in menopausal women have shown injections of testosterone to be well tolerated and safe.

Dr. Kaiser says that maybe someday soon there will be a testosterone formulation for women that will avoid some of the potential side effects, but she is reluctant to prescribe for females until then.

Testosterone: Pills or Shots?

Without the natural testosterone, men can develop intellectual slowing and abdominal obesity associated with heart disease, as well as decreased sexual function.

Dr. Kaiser says doctors can prescribe testosterone in pill form or injections: "Because the pills aren't absorbed efficiently in the body and may cause liver damage, we favor taking any needed testosterone by shot. The slight inconvenience of the needle seems outweighed by the increased effectiveness and safety of the drug." Usually, the shots must be given about every three weeks.

A new form of testosterone delivered in a tablet may improve sexual function without side effects in men with low testosterone, a John Hopkins study shows.[29]

"This is an easy way to administer a drug, and it was found to be safe and effective," says Dr. Dobs, the lead author. Results of the study, funded by the National Institutes of Health and Watson Pharmaceuticals, were presented June 12, 1996, at the International Congress of Endocrinology's annual meeting in San Francisco.

Thirteen men with low testosterone received a testosterone tablet that dissolves in the mouth or a placebo. Three months later, the men receiving the hormone tablets had normal sexual function and performed significantly better than those getting the placebo. The tablets allowed the men to perform as well sexually as when they received testosterone injections, but without prolonged exposure to a high hormone level caused by injections. The hormone level rises and drops steeply with injections, often causing mood swings and other side effects. Studies have shown that recently developed testosterone skin patches also deliver the hormone at a steady level for a long period.

Side Effects

The testosterone market will reportedly exceed $400 million in 1997. Given by injection or tablet, testosterone stimulates target tissues to develop normally in androgen-deficient men. It is used to treat eunuchs and male-hormonal-change symptoms, and for breast engorgement in nonnursing mothers and to treat breast cancer in women who are one to five years postmenopausal. Potential adverse reactions in women include acne, edema, oily skin, weight gain, hairiness, hoarseness, clitoral enlargement, changes in libido, flushing, sweating, and vaginitis with itching; in prepubescent males, premature epiphyseal closure, priapism, (see Glossary), growth of body and facial hair, phallic enlargement; in postpubescent males, testicular atrophy, scanty sperm, decreased ejaculatory volume, impotence, breast enlargement, and epididymitis; in both sexes, edema, gastroenteritis, nausea, vomiting, diarrhea, constipation, changes in appetite, bladder irritability, jaundice, liver toxicity, and high levels of calcium in the blood. Contraindicated in men with enlarged or cancerous prostates, carcinoma of the male breast, high levels of calcium in the blood, heart, liver, or kidney dysfunction, and in premature infants. Should be used cautiously in patients with diabetes or heart disease, and in those taking ACTH, corticosteroids, or anti-coagulants. It should be taken with food. Androgens can increase the effects of blood thinners. May also interact with many other medications, including oral contraceptives, making these medications less effective or increasing their side effects.[30]

Summing it up, researchers at St. Louis University, Johns Hopkins, and elsewhere are studying whether testosterone-replacement therapy may improve men's muscle mass and strength, bone density, cholesterol level, sense of well-being, cognitive function, and balance. Testosterone replacement therapy has been shown to improve sexual function in men with low testosterone.

"Compared to estrogen research, we're fifteen years behind in investigating the benefits of testosterone," says Johns Hopkins endocrinologist Dr. Dobs.

Cancer researchers in the Midwest reported that the sex hormone megestrol acetate, sold by Bristol-Myers Squibb Co. under the brand name Megace, stimulated the appetite and fostered weight gain in patients emaciated by cancer.

Testosterone, of course, is not the only hormonal factor in male sexual function. An estimated 50 percent of diabetics are impotent, which has to do with insulin metabolism. And, according to William Masters, M.D., the famed sex therapist of the Masters and Johnson Institute, St. Louis, Missouri, "Mental fatigue plays a large role in sexual disinterest and unresponsiveness in older persons. For men particularly, business concerns and a consequent sense of exhaustion with depressive elements may cast a pall on their personal life."[31]

Dr. Masters also points out other factors that may impinge on potency:

- Excessive consumption of food and alcohol
- Fear of failure

He wrote that androgen supplementation is not indicated for all older men solely for the tonic effects of enhanced body economy (increased libido, improved muscle tone, improved appetite, and higher energy levels). Androgens have only a temporary impact on sexual desire and responsiveness if the patient does not have a true hypoandrogenic state.

While most men wish to maintain their muscle strength and potency as long as possible, each man will have to decide for himself whether the benefits outweigh the risks.

8. ESTROGEN—SEXUAL DESIRE, DESIRABILITY, AND ABILITY

Avoiding Age-Associated Dysfunctions

There is a hormone—estrogen—that many eminent scientists today say prevents or delays such signs associated with aging as fragile bones, wrinkled skin, shrunken and flabby genitals, tooth loss, heart attacks, and even senility. Millions of mature women are taking it. Have they made a Faustian bargain?

In the German legend, a learned doctor, Faust, sold his soul to the devil in exchange for youth. Have many of today's post-menopausal women bargained for the promise of prolonged youth with estrogen replacement therapy (ERT) by risking illness and perhaps death from cancer or strokes? Have they been misled into taking this powerful hormonal supplement by pharmaceutical companies that reap billions from its sale, or is ERT a prime example of the priceless, long-sought youth elixir?

Conflicting reports regularly appear in the scientific literature, but the consensus today seems to be that for many postmenopausal women, hormone replacement therapy does everything promised, but for some others it is, indeed, a Faustian bargain.

In this chapter, the history and scientific reports of the benefits and consequences of female hormone replacement therapy are described. The aim is to help you make an informed choice with your physician about whether the anti-aging benefits of female hormone replacement therapy are a good bargain for you or your loved one.

THE POWER OF ESTROGEN

When God took a rib from Adam's side to make a woman, He must have added an extra ingredient because the female of the species is biologically stronger and longer lasting than the male. Although more human males are conceived, their attrition rate in the womb is higher—about 160 aborted or stillbirth males for every 100 females. In twin pregnancies, when male and female compete for survival, the female wins.

The life expectancy of the American woman has increased by 28.1 years since 1900, while the life span of the American male has lengthened only 24.1 years. Not surprisingly, females in the United States outnumber males. At ages fifty-five to sixty, there are 5,708 more women per 100,000 than men, and at ages seventy-five to eighty, there are 25,729 more women.[1]

What is that extra ingredient in women that makes them live longer? For a number of scientists, the answer is simple—the female hormone estrogen.

Estrogen does not exert its effects alone. It depends, first of all, upon the biologic responsiveness of the various female organs and, second, upon the presence of other hormones, particularly progesterone. Progesterone works during the second half of the menstrual cycle to create a lining in the uterus as a viable home for an egg, and to shed the lining if the egg is not implanted. Both estrogen and progesterone are produced by the ovaries in cyclic fashion in response to stimulation from the central nervous system.

A woman, in her entire lifetime, produces barely two table-spoonfuls of estrogen and progesterone, yet the survival of the human race depends upon the release and perfect synchronization of microscopic amounts of these substances.

The years between puberty—the onset of menstruation—and menopause—the cessation of it—are growing longer. The age at which menarche occurs has decreased by roughly four months every ten years since 1800, and there has been a corresponding increase in the age of women at the time of menopause.[2] The reason for this change is unclear, although early evidence points to better nutrition.

In most creatures the reproductive cycle and life itself are closely intertwined. When one ends, so does the other. Yet, today women in Western nations live almost as many years after menopause as before.

WHAT CAUSES MENOPAUSE?

For a yet unknown reason, in a woman's midthirties her ovaries begin to decline in hormone production. By her late forties, the process accelerates and her hormones fluctuate, causing her to have irregular menstrual cycles and unpredictable episodes of heavy bleeding. In her early to mid fifties, her periods cease entirely. However, her estrogen production does not completely stop. Her ovaries decrease their output significantly, but may still produce a small amount. Also, another form of estrogen is emitted from her fat tissue with help from her adrenal glands (above the kidneys). Although this form of estrogen is weaker than that produced by the ovaries, it increases with age and with the amount of fat tissue.

The fluctuation in female hormones affects other glands. The endocrine system must constantly readjust itself to work effectively. The hot flash—that sudden sensation of intense heat—appears to be a direct result of the endocrines emitting large amounts of hormones in an effort to restore the delicate balance.

Young women who have both their ovaries removed surgically experience an abrupt menopause and may have more distressing symptoms. Their hot flashes may be more severe, more frequent, and last longer. The women may have a greater risk of heart disease, osteoporosis, and depression. The reasons are not completely understood. When only one of their ovaries is removed, their menopause usually occurs naturally. When their uterus is removed and their ovaries remain, their menstrual periods stop but other menopausal symptoms, if any, usually occur at the same age that they would naturally.

Ovarian hormones also affect all other tissues including the breasts, vagina, bones, blood vessels, gastrointestinal tract, urinary tract, and skin. With advancing age, the walls of the vagina become thinner, dryer, less elastic, and more vulnerable to infection. These changes can make sexual intercourse uncomfortable.

The alterations in the urinary tract sometimes leave women more susceptible to involuntary loss of urine, particularly if certain chronic illnesses or urinary infections are also present. Exercise, coughing, laughing, lifting heavy objects, or similar movements put pressure on the bladder and may cause small amounts of urine to leak.

That mysterious biological clock inevitably reaches the hour when menses cease and the above-mentioned results occur. Can replacement of the diminished female hormones to premenopausal levels turn back the clock?

DISCOVERY OF THE "FEMALE PRINCIPLE"

Since 1931, when the first woman patient received a dose of the newly isolated female hormone estrogen, millions of women have received estrogen therapy for a variety of reasons: for birth control, menstrual problems, failure of ovaries to develop, and of course, for relief of the symptoms of menopause.

Evidence for the existence of estrogen came from observing what happened to subjects (animal and human) who had both ovaries removed. In 1900, a Viennese gynecologist, Dr. Emil Knauer, found that doing ovarian transplants prevented the symptoms associated with the loss of ovaries. Scientists searched for the "female principle" and eventually isolated the hormones that had such profound effects. Today we know a good deal more about their intricate formation and functioning. We know, for example, several parts of the brain as well as a number of glands such as the thyroid, parathyroid, pancreas, and adrenals are involved. Much research, however, remains to be done before these processes are thoroughly understood.

In the early 1980s, a Brooklyn gynecologist, Robert Wilson, M.D., did much to popularize the idea that estrogen was a youth exilir. In one of his first articles, he and Thelma A. Wilson, R.N., from the department of obstetrics and gynecology of Methodist Hospital, Brooklyn, New York, wrote in the *Journal of the American Geriatrics Society:*

"The unpalatable truth must be faced that all postmenopausal women are castrates. There is a variation in degree but not in fact. Men do not live as long as the so-called weaker sex. However, they age, if free from serious disease, in a proportional manner. The primary adrenal axis and thyroid are relatively intact until very old age. The gonads fade gradually, but there is no sudden shutdown."[3]

The Wilsons wrote, "In the past, so-called mental 'adjustment' to the 'change of life' was necessary. There was no choice. Without such adjustment, the ensuing years were hardly endurable. Today there are three choices: (1) make the best possible adjustment, (2) postpone the adjustment, or (3) avoid the necessity.

"Once aware of these choices, it is reasonably certain that most women will not choose either adjustment or postponement. Instead they will elect to avoid their probable fate—hypertension, arteriosclerosis, flabby breasts, dowager's hump, and atrophic genitals.

"Three things are virtually lacking in the untreated post-menopausal women: ova, estrogen, and progesterone. Ova cannot be purchased, but the two steroids can: lifelong substitution therapy is simply a matter of 'know-how.' There is a great need for the reorientation of almost every man and woman in the civilized world."

MEASURING ESTROGEN LEVELS

A lot has happened since the Wilsons wrote that. Ova can be purchased in the burgeoning infertility centers around the world, and women in their fifties and sixties can have their fertility revived artificially. But for millions of mature women, just having their estrogen restored to premenopausal levels to prevent signs associated with aging is enough.

Researchers have learned how to measure estrogen levels by observing the changes in every part of a woman's reproductive system during her menstrual cycle. It is now possible to take samples of tissues, cells, or secretions at different phases of the cycle and learn something about a woman's hormonal status. For example, one type of test is based on the series of changes that the endometrium, the lining of the uterus, undergoes in response to both estrogen and progesterone. By examining a bit of endometrial tissue under the microscope, a pathologist gains excellent information about hormone production and whether or not ovulation is occurring.

A second type of test uses the changes that occur in the cervical secretions during an ovulatory cycle as a basis for chemical and laboratory studies of hormone levels.

Knowledge of these changes in women who are menstruating

becomes important to physicians evaluating postmenopausal patients who are receiving estrogen.

WHAT ARE THE POTENTIAL ANTI-AGING BENEFITS OF FEMALE HORMONE REPLACEMENT THERAPY?

Restoration of more youthful levels of female hormones can not only alleviate the hot flashes and other discomforts of menopause but may, new research shows, prevent or postpone age-associated disabilities, as pointed out at the beginning of this chapter. Among the prime benefits of replacement therapy, according to pharmaceutical companies and many physicians, is estrogen's ability to keep bones from becoming fragile as we grow older.

Estrogen and Bones

Osteoporosis, the thinning of bone, is a major women's health problem. It is responsible for about 1.3 million fractures in the United States each year. About half a million women will fracture a vertebra, one of the bones that make up the spine, and about three hundred thousand will fracture a hip. Nationwide, treatment for osteoporotic fractures costs up to $10 billion per year. Vertebral fractures lead to curvature of the spine, loss of height, and pain. Between 12 and 20 percent of those who suffer a hip fracture do not survive the six months after the fracture.[4]

The condition of an older woman's skeleton depends on two things: the peak amount of bone attained before menopause and the rate of the bone loss thereafter. Hereditary factors are also important. Dietary calcium and vitamin D play a major part, but one of the biggest causes of bone loss is reported to be lack of estrogen. The loss of bone quickens during perimenopause, the transitional phase when estrogen levels drop significantly.

Scientists believe the best strategy for osteoporosis is prevention because currently available treatment only cuts bone loss in half and doesn't rebuild bone. Estrogen saves more bone tissue than even large daily doses of calcium. While it is boon for the bone, estrogen also affects all other tissues, and as you will read in this chapter, that can be a problem.

In a study performed at the University of Pittsburgh to determine the relationship between estrogen replacement therapy and fractures, 9,704 women, sixty-five years of age or older, participated. Those who used estrogen replacement were compared with women of the same age and situation who didn't. Estrogen was most effective in preventing hip fractures among those older than seventy-five. Current users who started estrogen within five years of menopause had a decreased risk for hip fractures, wrist fracture, and all nonspinal fractures when compared with women who had never used estrogen. Previous but discontinued use of estrogen for more than ten years had no substantial effect on the risk for fractures. The Pittsburgh researchers concluded that the current use of estrogen appears to decrease the risk of fracture in older women: "These results should suggest that for protection against fractures, estrogen should be initiated soon after menopause and continued indefinitely."[5]

Getting It in the Teeth

The benefit to bones of estrogen replacement therapy is reflected in tooth loss, according to two large studies in the mid-1990s.[6]

Tooth loss tends to increase with age. While the normal amount of teeth for adults is thirty-two, on average, adults under age forty-five lack three teeth, those ages forty-five to sixty-four are missing eleven teeth, and people over age sixty-five are missing sixteen teeth. About 40 percent of noninstitutionalized people over age sixty-five have no teeth.[7]

In a study of nearly four thousand women in a retirement

community in California, those who took estrogen were 36 percent less likely to have no teeth than women who didn't take hormones.

The author of the study, published in the *Archives of Internal Medicine* in 1995, Annlia Paganini-Hill, Ph.D., of the University of Southern California School of Medicine in Los Angeles, points out that women with severe osteoporosis are more than three times as likely as other women to lose their teeth, most likely because of loss of bone in the jaw that holds teeth in place.

"By preventing osteoporosis, estrogen-replacement therapy may be beneficial in preventing tooth loss and the need for dentures in older women," Dr. Paganini-Hill wrote. The California researcher acknowledged that the results need to be confirmed by other studies. For instance, if the estrogen users in the study tended to be healthier than the other women, they may have been less likely to lose their teeth regardless of whether they took hormone therapy, she points out.

Another study reported in the March 1996 issue of the *American Dental Association Journal* has added weight to the findings of Dr. Paganini-Hill. A Harvard-Brigham and Women's Hospital study asked 7,353 postmenopausal women if they had lost one or more teeth in 1990 and 1991. Researchers found that women who had used the female hormone regularly at some time were 24 percent less likely to lose their teeth than women who never took it.

Those currently using estrogen were 38 percent less likely to lose their teeth than nonusers. These researchers also said their work should be interpreted with caution because they didn't have any information about the dental health of the participants.

Older women and smokers using estrogen had only a slightly higher risk of tooth loss than those who were younger and did not smoke.

Estrogen and Heart Disease

The second most purported benefit of female hormone replacement therapy is against heart disease. Can hormone replacement therapy delay or prevent the number one killer of women over fifty years, heart disease? As pointed out earlier in this chapter, women do live longer than men. One of the major reasons is that they do not die of cardiovascular disease as early as men do. Females only start dying as fast or faster than males from heart disease after menopause.[8]

C. Noel Bairey Merz, M.D., medical director, Preventive and Rehabilitative Cardiac Center, Cedars-Sinai Medical Center, Los Angeles, is an enthusiastic advocate of estrogen replacement.[9] She points out that one out of two women over fifty will die of heart disease, and one out of five will get breast cancer. Of the breast cancer patients, only 2 to 3 percent will die of it.

She says estrogen sits on cell receptors for about fifty years, and then, over time, there is no estrogen and the arteries get out of control. She notes, "That's what causes a hot flash—the arteries dilate and contract because they are out of control."

She said studies have shown that in women with established heart disease, estrogen reduces the risk of a heart attack by 50 percent, while daily aspirin reduces the risk by 15 percent and ACE inhibitors (heart medications) by 25–30 percent.

A large new study of nurses has found that the combination pills, estrogen and progestin—taken in birth control pills and by women for menopause—are also highly effective against heart disease. The study, published in the *New England Journal of Medicine,* August 15, 1996, was based on sixteen years of follow-up of 59,337 women enrolled in the Nurses' Health Study.

Heart problems were rare in these women. There were just 770 documented heart attacks. Nevertheless, both kinds of hormone therapy appeared to help. The risk of heart disease was 61 percent lower in postmenopausal women taking the combination of hormones that in those who took no hormones, and it was 40 percent lower in those getting estrogen alone.[10]

While the figures suggested that combined hormones are just as good as straight estrogen for the heart, the study was not large enough to conclude the combination pills are actually better, according to the National Institutes of Health, which sponsored the study.

Estrogen and Longevity

One study reported in 1996 that ERT not only protects against heart disease but from dying in general. In the January 2, 1996, issue of the *Journal of Obstetrics and Gynecology,* it was reported that women who took ERT enjoyed a 46 percent reduction in the rate of death from all causes and even greater reductions in the death rate from cardiovascular disease.

The lead author of the report, Bruce Ettinger, M.D., says, "The benefit of long-term estrogen use is large and positive." Women who use this relatively inexpensive drug can substantially reduce their overall risk of dying prematurely.

Dr. Ettinger said the research evaluated the medical histories of 454 women born between 1900 and 1915 and compared the health outcomes of those who started therapy with those who didn't. About half of the group, 232, used estrogen therapy for at least a year starting in 1969. An age-matched group of nonusers totaled 222. Only women who were generally healthy at the start of the study were selected.

Among those women who didn't use estrogen therapy, eighty-seven died from all causes. Among the estrogen users, fifty-three died.

Dr. Ettinger said most of the benefit was connected to preventing heart attacks and strokes, the leading killers of women.

For coronary heart disease, estrogen users had a 60 percent reduction in mortality risk. For other cardiovascular problems, such as stroke, the estrogen users had a 73 percent reduction in mortality.

If estrogen is indeed the anti-aging hormone for the heart and blood vessels as Dr. Ettinger and many other researchers maintain, how does it do its work?

One major theory has to do with that artery-clogging, fatlike substance cholesterol. Cholesterol is essential for producing new cells and manufacturing certain hormones. It is delivered throughout the body by tiny packages made of fat and lipoproteins. Lipoproteins are flat, disklike particles produced in the liver and intestines and released into the bloodstream. There are basically two major types, high-density lipoproteins (HDLs) and low-density lipoproteins (LDLs). It is believed HDLs pick up cholesterol and bring it back to the liver for reprocessing. Some researchers believe HDLs may also remove excess cholesterol from fat-engorged cells, possibly even those in artery walls. Because HDLs clear cholesterol out of the system and high levels of it are associated with decreased risk of heart disease, HDL is often called "good cholesterol." An LDL package, on the other hand, is considered "bad" because it drops its contents along artery walls as it travels from the liver to body cells.

The National Institutes of Health's National Cholesterol Education Program guidelines say our total cholesterol should be below 200 mg/dl, LDL below 130, and HDL cholesterol should be above 35 mg/dl. So it is not only the total amount of cholesterol in your blood that is important, but which lipoprotein package is carting it around.

A great deal of evidence links elevated blood cholesterol levels to coronary heart disease. The bad LDL cholesterol appears to increase while good HDL cholesterol seems to decrease in postmenopausal women as a direct result of estrogen deficiency, and this, many say, may be the culprit behind the postmenopausal heart risk. There are concerns, however, about the long-term effects of the other female hormone, progesterone, used with estrogen for hormone replacement in postmenopausal women. Progesterone reportedly may raise harmful LDL while lowering beneficial HDL.[11]

Genes and Estrogen

Johns Hopkins researchers have another theory about the link between aging depletion of estrogen and heart disease. They believe, as a result of their study, that as some people age, their risk for coronary artery disease rises because a genetic change in their heart's blood vessels makes the vessels unable to benefit from estrogen. This is the first study to show that deactivation of the estrogen receptor gene occurs in cardiovascular tissue, the Hopkins scientists report. The process, called *methylation,* appears to cripple or weaken the tissue's response to the female hormone estrogen. Many studies indicate estrogen replacement therapy reduces heart disease risk by about 50 percent in postmenopausal women by improving blood flow to the heart.

"The findings are preliminary, but our ultimate goal is to help explain why some women respond better to estrogen replacement therapy and to find a way to prevent or reverse methylation in cardiovascular tissue," says Wendy S. Post, M.D., the study's lead author and a cardiology fellow. A drug to keep the gene active may reduce the risk of cardiovascular disease in some patients, she says.

The Hopkins investigators examined normal and diseased heart blood vessels and fatty deposits in the vessels in forty-one men and women over age thirty-seven. They found the gene had been inactivated by methylation to a greater extent in the diseased tissue than in the healthy tissue. The results suggest the gene may be inactivated in the atria (the heart's upper chambers) as a result of natural aging and contributes to atherosclerosis, a buildup of fatty deposits in the blood vessels to the heart, says Post.

It is unclear why methylation, which occurs differently in various tissues of the body, happens only in some people.

What if it is not the lack of estrogen that causes cardiovascular problems in postmenopausal women but the increase in the male hormone testosterone, as many other researchers maintain?

Investigators at the University of Texas Health Science Center at San Antonio hypothesize that in postmenopausal women decreased estrogen and testosterone would be associated with fat-clogged arteries and heart attack risk.[12] They tested the levels of sex hormones in 253 postmenopausal women not taking replacement hormones. The researchers found the level of estrogen was inversely associated only with the HDL-cholesterol/total-cholesterol ratio and that it was the testosterone increase in postmenopausal women that is associated with artery-clogging changes.

What about Sex?

Can replenishing female sex hormones restore sexual interest and performance?

Two-thirds of all married women in their sixties enjoy sex as much as they did when they were younger, according to a study by a gynecologist at the University of Medicine and Dentistry of New Jersey–Robert Wood Johnson Medical School.[13] Not only do most married women in their sixties desire sex, but they engage in it an average of five times a month, according to the study. But for some women, menopause brings a decrease in sexual activity. Reduced hormone levels cause subtle changes in genital tissue and are thought to be linked also to a decline in sexual interest. Lower estrogen levels decrease the blood supply to the vagina and the nerves and glands surrounding it. This makes delicate tissues thinner, drier, and less able to produce secretions to comfortably lubricate before and during intercourse. Estrogen creams and oral estrogen can restore secretions and tissue elasticity. Over-the-counter water-soluble lubricants can also help. Intravaginal administration of estriol prevents recurrent urinary tract infections in postmenopausal women, thereby removing another barrier to enjoyable sex.[14]

William H. Masters, M.D., of the famed Masters & Johnson Institute, St. Louis, Missouri, wrote in 1986 about sex, aging, and reality: "Continued sexual activity in later years not only helps maintain normal function but mitigates many of the involutional changes caused by sex steroid deprivation. By making patients aware of this important fact and of the altered responses and altered needs for stimulation that accompany aging, one can prevent the anxiety reactions that so often cause sexual dysfunction or abstinence."[15]

Skin

HRT seems to help preserve skin elasticity and thickness, much as Dr. Wilson maintained in 1983. It helps maintain the collagen that keeps skin looking plumped up and moist.

THE FAUSTIAN BARGAIN

So, female hormone replacement therapy can, it seems, ward off heart attacks, sagging genitals, wrinkled skin, lost teeth, senility, and other signs associated with aging including dry skin. But what about gallbladder disease, strokes, and cancer?

Getting Stoned—Gallbladder Problems

The gallbladder is a saclike organ, underlying the liver, in which bile, which helps to process fats, is stored, concentrated, and delivered to the digestive tract as needed. Stones (calculi) occur in the gallbladder in an estimated 25 percent of persons over age fifty.[16] Female hormone replacement doubles the incidence of gallbladder disease.[17] A proposed mechanism is that the estrogens decrease enzyme breakdown of the bile. Since bile is 75 to 90 percent saturated with cholesterol, this increase in biliary cholesterol may lead to precipitation and stone formation.

Strokes

It has been known for a long time that high doses of estrogen in early oral contraceptives were associated with blood clots. The effect appears to be dose related. Controlled epidemiologic studies of postmenopausal estrogen replacement have shown no increase in blood clots. In some women, estrogen replacement may lower blood pressure, and in some it may worsen high blood pressure.[18] The use of ERT in women with a family history of strokes, blood clots, or even migraine headaches is not recommended by most physicians, and in fact, the FDA requires that hormone replacement literature point out that large doses of estrogens, such as a 30-milligram daily dose to treat breast cancer, are linked to increased risk of heart attack and blood-clot conditions. (By comparison, the usual daily dosage for menopausal symptoms is 0.01 to 0.05 mg of ethinyl estradiol or 0.30 to 1.25 mg of conjugated estrogens.)[19]

Dr. Paganini-Hill, who is professor of preventive medicine at the University of Southern California, studied replacement therapy and stroke. She reported in *Progressive Cardiovascular Disease,* November-December 1995, that the results of nineteen studies reexamining the association between estrogen replacement therapy and cerebrovascular disease are inconsistent. She said, "Although all seven studies of death from stroke found a 20 percent to 60 percent reduction in risk among estrogen users relative to nonusers, studies of incident stroke and subarachnoid hemorrhage [in the brain] in particular are conflicting, with risks from 0 to 2.3. Although a protective effect of estrogen concerning stroke is biologically plausible, information regarding effects of dose, duration, and discontinuation of estrogen is limited and contradictory. Additionally, selection bias, recall bias, and confounding cannot be completely discounted. Further studies are needed to determine durations, and types of estrogen; the consequences of combined estrogen/progesterone regimens and other routes of administration; whether or not other factors (such as age and smoking) modify or confound estrogen's effect on stroke risk."

There is evidence from the large national Postmenopausal Estrogen/Progestin Interventions (PEPI) Trial as well as other studies, notably one involving more than twenty-three thousand women in Sweden, that HRT reduces the risk of stroke and does not raise blood pressure. Many physicians believe that the reason HRT does not cause the same vascular symptoms that birth control pills do is because the amount of estrogen in them is much lower than in the contraceptive combinations.

Dr. Howard Fillit, a professor of geriatrics, points out that blood clots reported in the past with estrogen use were related to estrogen in birth control pills, and high levels of progestin. Those oral compounds were ten times more potent than those in use today for HRT. Furthermore, he said, HRT products have a short half-life (they get out of the body quicker).[20]

Harvard University investigators wanted to determine whether past use of oral contraceptives and postmenopausal use of hormones influenced the incidence of blood clots in the veins or lungs. They sent questionnaires to 112,593 women every two years from 1976 to 1992. In 1976, the women were thirty to fifty-five. They reported there were 123 cases of primary blood clots to the lungs and that current users of postmenopausal hormones had an increased risk of two to one. However, past use showed no relationship to the blood clots. The researchers also found that current users of birth control pills had about twice the risk of nonusers but the statistics were based on only five women who used the pill who suffered blood clots to the lungs.

Dr. Francine Grodstein, the lead researcher, wrote that while the data suggests an increased risk of primary pulmonary embolism with current postmenopausal hormone use, the overall rate in healthy women was low.

"The many other substantial risks and benefits of hormone use observed in epidemiological studies including possible increase in endometrial and breast cancer and decreases in the rates of heart disease and osteoporosis, are more important factors to be considered by women choosing whether to use hormones after menopause," she concludes.[21]

What about Susceptibility to Cancer?

In the 1940s, when estrogen was first offered to menopausal women, it was given alone and in high doses. Today, after fifty years of trial and error, it is well known that estrogen stimulates growth of the inner lining of the uterus (endometrium), which sheds during menstruation. It increased the rate of endometrial cancer among women on estrogen replacement. Today, most doctors prescribe a lower dose of estrogen plus a synthetic progesterone, progestin, to counteract estrogen's dangerous effect on the uterus. Progestin reduces the risk of cancer by causing monthly shedding of the endometrium. The obvious drawback is that menopausal women resume monthly bleeding, something most women don't want to do. In addition, other unpleasant side effects of progestin often discourage women from continuing HRT. These include breast tenderness, bloating, abdominal cramping, anxiety, irritability, and depression.

Many reports have noted that ERT may increase the risk of uterine and breast cancer. In the February 1996 issue of the *Journal of the American Medical Association,* however, Howard Judd, M.D., chair of the Postmenopausal Estrogen/Progestin Interventions (PEPI) Trial, and his colleague wrote, "Although numerous investigations have reviewed endometrial [uterine lining] changes in women given estrogen plus a progestin, these studies have been flawed by design issues related to lack of proper controls, limited sample sizes, and short follow-up periods."

The PEPI Trial involved several research centers and hundreds of volunteers. One group of women was given estrogen alone, another a placebo, and a third group estrogen and progestin (a combination reported to counteract the effect of estrogen alone on the uterine lining).

The women were meticulously followed over three years. Of the 119 women who received estrogen alone, 74 developed some type of endometrial tissue overgrowth, a potential precursor to uterine cancer. Of 118 in an estrogen-progestin group, only 6 developed the overgrowth, and only 2 of 199 women in the placebo group developed the condition. Women who have had the uterus surgically removed have no risk of endometrial cancer.

Many physicians have concluded that with concurrently administered progestin, the risk of endometrial cancer is less than that in untreated postmenopausal women.[22]

Estrogen and Colon Cancer

Colon cancer is the third most common type of cancer. Only lung cancer and breast cancer are more common. Men and women are equally susceptible to this cancer of the large intestine, which is most prevalent among people over forty, and especially among those who are in their sixties and seventies. A large study released in April 1996 found that estrogen users had a 29 percent lower risk of dying from colon cancer than nonusers. For those on estrogen more than 10 years, the risk was 55 percent lower. Dr. Eugenia E. Calle of the American Cancer Society, the lead author of the study, maintained that estrogen may have a beneficial effect on bile acids or on the lining of the colon. She said her findings are consistent with the other reports suggesting a protective role of estrogen replacement in the development of colorectal cancer. Thus, she says, the potential estrogen-colorectal cancer protective effects merit further investigation.[23]

Ovarian Cancer

An American Cancer Society study of 240,000 women found that those who took estrogen for at least six years had a 40 percent increased risk of fatal ovarian cancer. For those taking estrogen for eleven years or more, the risk was 70 percent higher than for women who had never used ERT.[24]

Previous studies of ERT and ovarian cancer have been inconclusive, according to Carmen Rodriguez, an epidemiologist for the American Cancer Society and principal investigator of the study. She said this study, first of all, is prospective, meaning that information is gathered before cancer occurs. This technique eliminates the possibility that the women's recollection of ERT use was triggered by their diagnosis with cancer. In addition, the study is large, and researchers were able to adjust their data for many known and possible ovarian cancer risk factors. Finally, a large number of women had used ERT for many years, allowing researchers to examine risk by duration of use.

Rodriguez said, however, that the results should be interpreted cautiously: "The findings from this study may not apply to women using ERT today because the normal dose is generally less than that prescribed when women in the study were being treated. Also, current standard hormone replacement therapy includes progesterone, which was uncommon in the 1970s and 1980s."

Breast Cancer

The addition of progestins to estrogen therapy does not reduce the risk of breast cancer among postmenopausal women. The substantial increase in the risk of breast cancer among older women who take hormones suggests that the trade-offs between risks and benefits should be carefully assessed.

Graham Colditz, M.B., B.S., and his colleagues at Harvard Medical School reported in the *New England Journal of Medicine,* June 1995, that women using hormone replacement had a higher risk of breast cancer than women who had never used the therapy. Based on an ongoing evaluation of more than 121,000 women, researchers found the risk was most pronounced in women over fifty-five who have used HRT for at least five years. It appears that the combined hormones may put women at a higher risk for breast cancer than does estrogen alone.[25]

A month after the *New England Journal of Medicine*'s report, a *Journal of the American Medical Association* report concluded that HRT does not seem to increase a middle-aged woman's risk of breast cancer. The study questioned more than one thousand women between the ages of fifty and sixty-four. The *JAMA* report noted that using combined therapy for more than eight years was associated with, if anything, a reduction in the risk of breast cancer. The researchers, from the Division of Public Health Sciences, Fred Hutchinson Cancer Research Center, Seattle, Washington, did caution, "Nonetheless, since the use of combined estrogen-progestin HRT has only recently become prevalent, future investigations must assess whether breast cancer incidence is altered many years after estrogen-progestin HRT has been initiated, particularly among long-term users."[26]

Oral contraceptives contain higher doses of estrogen and progestins than replacement pills. British epidemiologists, who collected data on 53,297 women with breast cancer and 100,239 women without breast cancer from fifty-four studies conducted in twenty-five countries, came to the following conclusion: "Women who are currently using combined oral contraceptives or have used them in the past ten years are at a slightly increased risk of having breast cancer diagnosed, although the additional cancers diagnosed tend to be localized to the breast. There is no evidence of an increase in the risk of having breast cancer diagnosed ten or more years after cessation of use, and the cancers diagnosed then are less advanced clinically than the cancers diagnosed in never-users."[27]

Women who have a family history of breast cancer and who ever used estrogen replacement therapy had a significantly higher risk than those who had not, according to a meta-analysis by researchers from the Center for Environmental Health and Injury Control and the School of Public Health, Emory University, Atlanta, Georgia.[28]

One issue that troubles many physicians is the use of HRT in survivors of breast cancer.[29] Several studies have shown reduced breast cancer recurrence rates in such patients who have received estrogen replacement. Nevertheless, physicians are reluctant to prescribe the hormone since many breast cancers are estrogen sensitive.

The FDA requires that hormone replacement products carry a warning against their use by women who have had cancer.

If you have a family history of breast cancer, you would be wise to discuss hormone replacement therapy thoroughly with your physician and decide for yourself if you wish to make a potential "Faustian bargain."

CHOICES OF HORMONE REPLACEMENT

The Food and Drug Administration says estrogen prescriptions in the United States more than doubled between 1982 and 1992. About a quarter of U.S. women at or past menopause—roughly 10 million—take the hormone. Premarin, an estrogen replacement medication, is the number one prescription drug in the United States.[30] As baby boomers approach menopause, the biological clock that causes menopause will strike for 30 million of them in the next eight years.

Examples of Available Therapies

Hormone therapy relieves the discomfort of hot flashes in most cases. Some women find relief in herbal preparations or vitamin E, and some women do not need any substances to counteract their mild symptoms of menopause. In both men and women, estrogen helps stabilize the opening and closing of blood vessels. Women manufacture most estrogens in the ovaries and adrenal glands, with increases during pregnancy from the placenta. Men produce low levels of estrogen in the testes. Fat cells also may produce estrogen.

One of the problems with hormone replacement therapy, according to Gerson Weiss, M.D., professor of obstetrics and gynecology at the University of Medicine and Dentistry of New Jersey–University Hospital, Newark, is compliance.[31]

"Women stay on it for less than a year. Primarily because of abnormal bleeding and fear of breast cancer," he says, and adds that newer routines such as continuous low doses of estrogen and progestin instead of the on-and-off routines of the past will ameliorate the abnormal bleeding problem.

Therapeutic estrogens made synthetically or derived from pregnant mare's urine are formulated as oral, injectable, vaginal, or stick-on patches.

Examples:

Estrogens, conjugated—Premarin. Progens. A mixture of estrogens obtained from natural sources. Used to prevent post-menopausal osteoporosis.

Estrone—Theelin. An estrogen used to treat atrophic vaginal inflammation, primary failure of the ovaries, symptoms of menopause, cancer of the prostate, and to prevent osteoporosis.

Estraderm—A transdermal preparation used to treat menopausal symptoms and/or to prevent osteoporosis. The Estraderm system releases through the skin small amounts of estradiol, a female hormone made by the ovaries.

Nonpharmaceutical Products

In addition to prescription hormone replacement therapy there are the over-the-counter products and foods that contain phytoestrogens—plant estrogens. Although they are considerably less active than those in animals, habitual exposure may lead to the accumulation of levels that are active in humans. Dr. Leon Bradlow of the Strang-Cornell Cancer Research Lab, New York, has explored how plant chemicals influence estrogen metabolism and thus how a diet high in fruits and vegetables might inhibit breast cancer.[32] Scientists know that estradiol, the precursor to estrogen, can take one of two metabolic pathways in the body turning into either a 16-hydroxylated form or a 2-hydroxylated form of estrogen. The 16-form is stimulatory and more dangerously reactive. Women with a high risk of breast cancer have elevated levels of the 16-form in their blood. Tissue from breast tumors contains more of the 16-form of estrogen, researchers have found, than does surrounding noncancerous breast tissue. The 2-form of estrogen is relatively inert and has been found to be elevated in women who are vigorous athletes and in those who eat many cruciferous vegetables (see Glossary). Phytoestrogens—isoflavones, genistein, and daidzein—are contained in soy products and may be one reason Orientals, who eat a lot of soy, have a much lower rate of breast and prostate cancers. Cabbage-family vegetables also contain the phytoestrogen genistein, which seems to block the growth of new blood vessels, essential for some tumors to grow and spread. Sheep grazing on some clovers are prone to reproductive failure because of genistein in the plants. Soybeans contain both plant estrogens and progesterones. Mexican yams, from which popular contraceptive pills are made, contain plant estrogens. For example:

Natural progesterone cream contains wild-yam extract, progesterone, chamomile, burdock-root extract, black-cohosh-root extract, Siberian-ginseng extract, almond oil, jojoba oil, safflower oil, avocado oil, aloe vera gel, and vitamin E. The user is instructed to apply one-fourth to three-fourths of a teaspoon to soft tissue—abdomen, inner thighs, buttocks—twice a day or as needed. It is advertised as stimulating the body's natural production and regulation of estrogen, progesterone, testosterone, and other hormones.

POTENTIAL SIDE EFFECTS OF HORMONE REPLACEMENT THERAPY

Roughly 10 percent of women who use estrogen experience side effects. Check with your doctor as soon as possible if any of the following estrogen side effects occur:

- Swollen feet and lower legs
- Rapid weight gain
- Breast pain
- Increased breast size
- Blood-filled skin sores
- Changes in vaginal bleeding

- Confusion
- General feeling of illness
- Joint or muscle aches
- Breast lumps or discharge from nipples
- Mental depression
- Persistent nausea or vomiting
- Pains in the stomach, side, or abdomen
- Sores in the mouth or nose or on lower legs, thighs, forearms, genitals, soles, or palms
- Uncontrolled jerky muscle movement
- Unusual tiredness
- Yellow eyes or skin

Patients who develop new health problems or have questions should check with their doctor.

People taking estrogens should get emergency medical help if any of the following symptoms of blood clots occur:

- Sudden or severe headache
- Sudden loss of coordination
- Sudden loss or change of vision
- Pains in the chest, groin, or leg, especially in the calf
- Sudden, unexplained shortness of breath
- Sudden slurring of speech
- Weakness or numbness in an arm or leg

Side effects that may require non-emergency medical care if severe or bothersome include mild acne, stomach bloating, appetite loss, overgrowth of the gums, problems wearing contact lenses due to dry eyes, and migraine headaches. Exposure to the sun can cause brown, blotchy skin spots, so it's wise to use sunscreen. Some patients may have other side effects.

Estrogens may affect certain diagnostic laboratory tests, such as the glucose tolerance test, so it's important that patients using estrogens tell the doctor or laboratory personnel performing the procedure.

UNANSWERED QUESTIONS

The Women's Health Initiative (WHI) is the largest prevention study ever funded by the National Institutes of Health.[33] It has already enrolled 27,500 for the hormone trial for women fifty to seventy-nine. The study is assessing the long-term benefits and risks of hormone therapy for cardiovascular disease, osteoporosis, and breast and uterine cancer. It will also help determine the effects of calcium supplementation, dietary changes, and exercise in women in this age group. Women with a uterus will receive estrogen in combination with progestin or an inactive pill. Women without a uterus will receive estrogen alone or an inactive pill.

Participants are placed in groups by chance, thereby eliminating any possibility that differences in health characteristics of the groups will account for any subsequent difference in health outcomes. The participants will be followed for an average of nine years. At the conclusion of this trial—first results are expected in about 2005—scientists will know more certainly whether estrogen lowers heart disease and bone fracture rates or increases breast cancer rates. The effects of adding progestin to estrogen will also be known. Then for the first time, armed with conclusive data, doctors will be able to answer more accurately the Faustian bargain questions—are the benefits worth the risks in anti-aging female hormone replacement? It is a multicenter, prospective, longitudinal, randomized trial comparing hormone replacement therapy with placebo and may eventually address many of the unanswered questions such as:

- How long is estrogen effective for each system of the body—bones, heart, blood vessels, nervous, endocrine?
- What is the best dose and route of administration of estrogen and progestin to prevent side effects yet maintain efficacy?
- How long is estrogen safe to take?
- When should you stop estrogen? Seventy or eighty years?
- Does estrogen act the same way in older women as in younger women?
- Are there effective alternatives to HRT?
- Who will benefit from hormone replacement therapy and is it possible to identify those individuals prospectively?
- What is the relationship between hormone replacement therapy and the initiation or exacerbation of breast cancer?
- Would a seventy-five-year-old woman with an intact uterus need progestins to protect an organ that is unlikely to develop endometrial cancer over her lifetime of use?

Preliminary data from the PEPI study reported in the *Journal of the American Medical Association,* December 16, 1994, showed that a large proportion of women with a uterus who received estrogen developed an overgrowth of the lining of the uterus that could lead to cancer. Early in 1995, PEPI had also reported that estrogen and estrogen with progestin improved some risk factors for heart disease. The WHI is testing directly whether these hormones will reduce the rate of heart disease in post-menopausal women.

While gynecologists acknowledge the risks of estrogen therapy, they tend to emphasize the pluses. "The benefits of HRT will outweigh the risks for most women," says Dr. William Andrews, former president of the American College of Obstetrics and Gynecology. "Eight times as many women die of heart attacks as die of breast cancer."[34]

SHOULD YOU OR SHOULDN'T YOU?

Despite conflicting findings, many physicians recommend HRT because in women over age sixty, the risks of heart disease and osteoporosis are greater than those of breast, uterine, or ovarian cancer.

Heart disease is the leading cause of death among older women, but a woman can decrease her risk by as much as 35 percent with HRT, and the therapy can decrease the risk of bone fractures by 25 percent.

Dr. Isaac Schiff, chief of obstetrics and gynecology at Massachusetts General Hospital, puts it bluntly: "Basically, you are presenting women with the possibility of increasing the risk of getting breast cancer at age sixty in order to prevent a heart attack at age seventy and a hip fracture at age eighty. How can you make a decision like that for a patient?"[35]

Dr. Paganini-Hill, clinical professor of preventive medicine at the University of Southern California, who is too young to take ERT, said she would hesitate to take it if she had a family history of breast cancer.

"On the other hand, if I also had a family history of heart disease, I would, because the benefits outweigh the risks," she says.[36]

Women live longer than their great-grandmothers. At the turn of the century, women died before or shortly after their ovaries shut down so they never had to face heart attacks, hip fractures, and high cholesterol.

Fran E. Kaiser, M.D., associate director of geriatric medicine at St. Louis University Medical School, says that every women has to decide for herself, based upon her family history, her current risk factors, and her physician's advice. She should have a normal mammogram, a pelvic exam, and a lipid (blood fat) profile before she takes ERT.

Dr. Kaiser, who says she takes ERT herself, notes, "Estrogen has a positive, protective effect on the heart. Playing the odds may help make a decision about ERT: one out of two women after menopause have the risk of a heart attack, while one out of nine to twelve have the risk of breast cancer."

Your Risk Evaluation

To decide whether hormone replacement therapy is a good anti-aging bargain for you, you have to consider your personal risk factors. Growing older is, in itself, a risk factor, but you have to decide with the help of your physician whether you wish to play the odds.[37]

Heart Disease Risk Factors

- Smoking
- History of heart attack, stroke, and high blood pressure in close blood relatives
- Elevated total blood cholesterol (above 240 mg/dl is high; 200 to 239 "borderline")
- HDL (good cholesterol) below 35

Osteoporosis Risk Factors

- Being of European or Asian origin. African-American women are at lower risk.
- Family history of osteoporosis
- Poor diet, especially one high in sodium and low in vitamins and minerals, particularly vitamin D and calcium
- Sedentary lifestyle, especially lack of weight-bearing exercise
- Obesity
- Smoking
- Heavy alcohol use
- Long-term use of certain medications such as cortisone or thyroid hormones

Breast Cancer Risk Factors

- A first-degree relative (mother or sister or aunt) with breast cancer
- Early onset of menstruation (before thirteen years) and/or late menopause (after fifty years)
- Not having had children, or having a first child after thirty-five
- Not having breast-fed
- Obesity
- A breast biopsy that suggested increased risk

Other Risk Factors

- If you might be pregnant. Estrogen therapy during pregnancy has been associated with an increased risk of birth defects, such as defects in the reproductive organs.
- If you have or have had cancer
- If you follow a special diet or ever had an unusual or allergic response to estrogen or to foods, dyes, or preservatives
- If you have a family history of bone disease, endometriosis (in which endometrial tissue becomes implanted elsewhere), epilepsy, fibroids, gallbladder disease, heart or circulatory disease, stroke, kidney disease, liver disease, migraine headaches, or excess calcium in the blood

Generally Not Recommended If

- You have an immediate family member—mother, sister, or daughter—who has had breast cancer
- If you have had a stroke
- If you have high blood pressure that is poorly controlled by medication
- If you suffer from migraine headaches
- If you have had circulatory problems such as a deep-vein blood clot

- If you have a family history of heart disease
- If you take other prescription or over-the-counter medicine. Estrogens may alter the effect of some other drugs, including drugs to prevent blood clots, diabetes drugs, calcium supplements, and a breast-cancer drug, tamoxifen.

In consultation with your physician, use the following to help you make up your mind whether you or a loved one should use female hormone replacement therapy.[38] Here is a summary of the pros and cons:

Pro

- HRT and ERT reduce the risk of osteoporosis.
- HRT and ERT relieve hot flashes.
- HRT and ERT reduce the risk of heart disease.
- HRT and ERT may improve mood and psychological well-being.
- HRT and ERT help prevent dryness and thinness of the skin associated with aging.
- HRT and ERT protect against gynecological and urological problems including infections and painful intercourse.
- HRT and ERT may delay or prevent the senility of Alzheimer's and vascular dementia (blocked blood vessels in the brain).

Con

- ERT increases the risk of endometrial cancer. (If you have had a hysterectomy, you can use estrogen alone since combination therapy is used to protect women against uterine cancer.)
- HRT and ERT may or may not increase the risk of breast and ovarian cancer. Long-term use may pose the greatest risk.

- HRT can have unpleasant side effects such as bloating or irritability.
- HRT and ERT may be dangerous for women susceptible to blood clots.

SUMMING UP

Only in this century have so many women lived beyond reproductive age. Cultural upheavals in industrial nations have made reproduction an option and the ending of reproductive capacity a crisis of aging. A woman's hormone levels change during menopause and beyond with multiple potential symptoms. Treatment with hormones can ameliorate these symptoms and potentially decrease the risk for the long-term consequences of menopause. Objective scientific data for absolutes regarding hormone replacement therapy are lacking, but increasingly, this epoch in the physical and emotional life of a woman is being defined by new cultural expectations.

Eventually, the decision to treat rests with each women and her physician.

9. AIDING BRAIN FUNCTION AND BRIGHTENING MOOD

Earlier in this book, the exquisite interactions between the brain, nerves, and endocrine systems were described. Is it any wonder then that scientists are trying to prevent or slow the aging of the brain with therapeutic hormone dosages? They are hoping that new understanding of how hormones in and out of the brain work may one day lead to means of preventing or reversing the forgetfulness and perhaps even the senility of old age.

Recently published research purports that the sex hormones—estrogen and testosterone—when given to persons in middle age and beyond can protect the brain from Alzheimer's, that memory-destroying disease, and act as anti-aging hormones for the brain.

Howard Fillit, M.D., clinical professor of geriatrics and corporate medical director for Medicare at NYLcare Plans, New York, points out, "We know it takes a long time for bone density to decline—about thirty years until the point that a person fractures a hip, for example. What about thirty years having the brain deficient in estrogen?"

Several studies recently published seem to show that women who take estrogen after menopause have less of a chance of developing Alzheimer's. In a study of 1,124 elderly women published August 17, 1996, in the British medical journal *Lancet,* Columbia-Presbyterian researchers in New York reported that only 5.8 percent of women who had taken estrogen developed Alzheimer's, compared with 16.3 percent of women who had not used it.

With each passing year of the five-year study, only 2.7 percent of the women who had used estrogen developed Alzheimer's as against 8.4 percent of those who had not used it. Moreover, the longer the women took estrogen, the lower their risk.

Black and white and Hispanic women benefited equally from estrogen, as did women of varying educational and socioeconomic levels.[1]

Neil Buckholtz, M.D., of the National Institute on Aging, Bethesda, Maryland, said that the findings are potentially the most promising advance ever made toward the prevention of Alzheimer's.[2]

Earlier, a similar report came from the Baltimore Longitudinal Study of Aging (BLSA) at Johns Hopkins School of Medicine. Under National Institute of Aging grants, the BLSA has been tracking a group of area residents for thirty-eight years for an investigation of normal aging.

Johns Hopkins neurologist Claudia Kawas, M.D., and her colleagues at Johns Hopkins and the NIA examined the records of 514 postmenopausal women or perimenopausal women who were followed up for as many as sixteen years. They found the women who had taken estrogen had a 54 percent reduction in risk for Alzheimer's compared with women who had never taken the hormones.[3]

Even when women who do take estrogen replacement develop Alzheimer's, evidently their progression of symptoms is slower than those who do not take the hormone. Several small trials have indicated that estrogen improves memory for postmenopausal women. And a tantalizing study, reported in 1993, found HRT enhanced the mental function of women with mild to moderate symptoms of Alzheimer's.

A Japanese study headed by T. Ohkura was designed to investigate the therapeutic efficacy of estrogen in female patients with dementia of the Alzheimer's type.[4] Of the fifteen women in the trial, the dementia of four was diagnosed as mild, seven as moderate, and four as severe. The effects of estrogen were evaluated by various psychological and psychometric assessments. It was found that ERT significantly improves cognitive functions, dementia symptoms, regional cerebral blood flow, and EEG activity in female patients with Alzheimer's. The study was reported in the *Journal of Endocrinology* in 1994.

Annlia Paganini-Hill, Ph.D., and her colleagues at the University of Southern California (USC), hypothesized that oral estrogen replacement would be less common among elderly women meeting the criteria of Alzheimer's disease than among nondemented elderly. In a case control study of estrogen replacement therapy, age and education were taken into consideration. When cognitive functions were compared between estrogen users and nonusers with Alzheimer's, the duration of dementia symptoms was an additional control. The study was done at USC, in Los Angeles, with women recruited from the community. The Alzheimer's patients were found to be less likely to use estrogen replacement, but the groups did not differ with regard to the total number of prescription medications taken or to the most frequently prescribed class of drug (thyroid medication). In patients with dementia, those using estrogen did not differ significantly from those not using estrogen in terms of age, education, or symptom duration, but their mean performance on cognitive screen instrument was significantly better. Conclusions consist with contentions that postmenopausal estrogen replacement therapy may be associated with a decreased risk of Alzheimer's and that estrogen replacement may improve cognitive performance of women with this illness.[5]

Dr. Paganini-Hill and her group, in cooperation with the University of Indiana and the University of California at Los Angeles, at this writing, were beginning a study of women with early or moderate Alzheimer's living in the community who were not taking estrogen. They will be given estrogen for four months, then the results will be evaluated by the university experts.[6]

ESTROGEN AND THE BRAIN

Just how estrogen works in the brain remains obscure, though research by Bruce McEwen, Ph.D., at Rockefeller University has shown that the hormone increases the number of connections between nerve cells in the hippocampus, a region that helps govern memory. Certain differences between female and male sexual behavior are programmed prenatally by the influence of estrogen or testosterone on the hypothalamus, a brain structure that also regulates temperature. Estrogen also increases the production of acetylcholine, a brain chemical that is abnormally low in Alzheimer's patients.

Researchers have found that the cholinergic neurons (see Glossary) of the brain have numerous estrogen receptors, and they occur on the same nerve cells that have receptors for nerve growth factor (see page 209); that estrogen in animals boosts levels of the nerve growth factor; and that estrogen injected in rats' brains strongly affects nerve cells in the cerebral cortex and the hippocampus—regions of the brain affected by Alzheimer's. These pieces of evidence have given rise to the theory that nerve growth factor and estrogen interact in some way to protect cholinergic nerve cells from degenerating.[7]

Frank Bellino, M.D., of the National Institute on Aging, who oversees grants for the study of menopause, says that until fairly recently, it was believed that it was strictly the ovary that caused women to go through menopause.[8]

"We now know that the hypothalamus and the pituitary play a part in menopause, and when we better understand why menopause occurs, then we will know more about this effect on bone loss, cardiovascular problems, and perhaps Alzheimer's," he says.

Dr. Fillit says estrogen also has an effect on inflammation and blood vessels, and new research is showing that inflammation may play a large part in the development of brain deterioration such as that seen in Alzheimer's and multiple vascular dementia. In addition to reducing inflammation, estrogen, Dr. Fillit points out, can

- Modulate neurotransmitter systems (messages sent between brain cells).
- Improve blood flow.
- Alter cytokine IL-2, a substance associated with inflammation released by cells.

Dr. Fillit points out that estrogen may help protect against vascular dementia over age eighty. It was once referred to as "hardening of the arteries" but is now believed to be a blood vessel disease in the brain that causes dementia.

Dr. Fillit believes that estrogen replacement therapy can delay the onset of Alzheimer's by five years. He points out that Alzheimer's currently costs $90 billion a year, and if it can be delayed even five years, it would be a tremendous saving to families and to society.[9]

Both men and women have estrogen receptors throughout the brain, including some areas affected by Alzheimer's. The hormone also appears necessary to maintain the integrity of a region of the hippocampus that is linked with memory changes associated with aging and Alzheimer's.[10]

Scientists from Oregon State University (OSU) are studying the role of estrogen as a possible therapeutic aid in postponing the development of Alzheimer's and other dementias.[11]

Certain estrogens have been shown to lower levels of apolipoprotein E (apoE), which normally helps transport cholesterol in the blood. A rare form of apoE, known as allele-type 4, is found in 50 to 60 percent of Alzheimer's patients, the researchers say.

"Postmenopausal females have much higher levels of senile dementia of the Alzheimer's type than do males," said Douglass J. Stennett, Ph.D., a professor of pharmacy at OSU. It may be that some women become more susceptible to dementia after menopause, when their bodies quit producing estrogen, leading to higher levels of apoE, a type of protein found to be inherited and related to Alzheimer's. One form of inherited apoE is found in those with early-onset Alzheimer's and another form with inherited late-onset Alzheimer's.[12]

The OSU scientists are working with cultures of nerve cells in a laboratory, trying to quantify the levels of apoE produced. They are then going to expose those cells to various forms of estrogen to see if levels of apoE, especially type 4, decrease. If they are successful, Dr. Stennett said, the next step will be to test the effect on postmenopausal women.

"We don't know whether this will work clinically," Stennett said. "It's too early to jump on the bandwagon. But if we can help postpone the onset of the disease, if we can buy these people a few more years, it may make the difference between allowing patients to stay at home with family or moving to a nursing home."

He points out that other researchers around the country are

trying a variety of methods to combat dementia. Those efforts include the use of anti-inflammatory drugs and antioxidants, such as vitamin E, which may protect the brain from damage by free radicals.

"Estrogen may be one of the most effective ways to reduce apoE," Dr. Stennett says. "It's also convenient, a large number of patients take it, and it's a relatively nontoxic drug."

He points out that it is difficult to get drugs into the brain because of the blood-brain barrier. Elderly patients don't always metabolize and excrete drugs at the same rate. If a drug already out there that is effective in lowering apoE type 4 can be found, it will be a whole lot easier than developing a new drug.

Alzheimer's is particularly frustrating, Dr. Stennett says, because it cannot be diagnosed for certain until after death. Instead, scientists call common symptoms "senile dementia of the Alzheimer's type."

Dr. Stennett said he experienced the devastation caused by the disease when one of his relatives went from a vigorous, full-of-life tennis player to helpless resident of a nursing home in two years.

"Early symptoms aren't easy to diagnose," he said. "Simple forgetfulness isn't a cause for alarm, but progressive memory lapses can indicate dementia. The short-term memory goes first, then the memory that's further back. You see people thinking in terms of years back. They may see their daughter and not recognize her or think she actually is their sister from fifty years ago, or even their mother."

Stennett, who works with Alzheimer's patients at Corvallis Manor Nursing Home, said the symptoms can progress rapidly or slowly. "It can get so bad that people literally can't find their way out of the bedroom to get to the kitchen."

The average life span of someone diagnosed with senile dementia of the Alzheimer's type is seven years, Stennett said. Some patients die within a year or two; others last fifteen years.

"The burden on a family can be enormous," Stennett said. "That's why delaying the onset of Alzheimer's for even a few years could be an enormous boon, emotionally and financially."

The OSU scientist and his colleagues are growing cultures of nerve cells in a laboratory to try to quantify the levels of apoE produced. They then will expose those cells to various forms of estrogen to see if levels of apoE decrease.

If they are successful, Stennett said, the next step will be to test the effect on postmenopausal women.[13]

Dr. Howard Fillit, a geriatrician and clinical professor of geriatrics at New York City's Mount Sinai Medical Center, has conducted small-scale tests of estrogen with women who have mild to moderate Alzheimer's. Patients who did not know the month or year could recall them after just three weeks on daily doses of hormones. The women became more alert, ate and slept better, and showed improved social behavior. Fillit believes testosterone therapy may prove equally useful for male patients. Estrogen is not yet an approved therapy for Alzheimer's, but as the evidence builds, it is fast becoming one of the brightest hopes in a so far bleak field.

At this writing, the Alzheimer's Disease Cooperative Study Unit was starting enrollment for an estrogen trial for women with mild Alzheimer's symptoms, which will examine how patients who take the drug for one year fare compared with women who receive a placebo.

What about Men?

Men may be at a lower risk for dementia because of an enzyme called aromatase, which converts testosterone to estrogen in the brain.[14] But just as some researchers have found that estrogen has a potential benefit for older women's brains, Johns Hopkins scientists are studying testosterone-replacement therapy for the same purpose in older men. The Baltimore researchers report that the primary male sex hormone may affect some learning skills, including improving visual and perceptual abilities in men. The findings may provide additional insight into testosterone's role in the brain.[15]

"This is interesting, early finding and it highlights the importance of studying the effects of sex hormones on brain function," says Adrian Dobs, M.D., senior author and an associate professor of medicine.

Results of the study, funded by the National Institutes of Health, were presented June 14, 1996, at the International Congress of Endocrinology's annual meeting in San Francisco. Ten men with low testosterone underwent word, memory, coordination, and other learning tests while on and off testosterone treatment. When receiving testosterone, they had improved visual and spatial skills and a better "mental grasp of objects"—fitting building blocks into the correct spaces, identifying pictures, and remembering shapes, patterns, and locations, the results showed. When not receiving testosterone, the men showed improved verbal fluency and verbal memory—making up sentences, defining words, and recalling words from a test.

This finding is interesting in view of an earlier German study published in 1991 in the *International Journal of Neuroscience*.[16] Marianne Hassler from the University of Tubingen's Department of Psychology, tested the testosterone levels of artistically talented persons. She said that certain kinds of giftedness, particularly artistic, musical, or mathematical talent, may have a hormonal basis, according to a number of studies between 1982 and 1987. Musical composers, instrumentalists, and painters were compared with nonmusicians from a student and from a nonstudent population on testosterone levels in saliva. Male composers had significantly lower mean testosterone values than male instrumentalists and male nonmusicians; female composers had significantly higher mean testosterone values than female instrumentalists and female nonmusicians. Painters of both sexes did not differ significantly from controls. Spatial ability was assessed in the five groups. Significant differences on spatial test performance were not reflected in differences on salivary testosterone.

Hassler concluded from the study that musical composers of both sexes were physiologically highly androgynous. Creative musical behavior was associated with testosterone levels that minimized sex differences.

And three years earlier than the Hassler studies, Doreen Kimura, Ph.D., a psychology professor at the University of Western Ontario, reported the effects of estrogen and the ability to perform tasks at various times of the month.[17] In two studies involving two hundred women, Dr. Kimura and graduate student Elizabeth Hampson found that the subjects performed better on tasks involving verbal skill or muscular coordination when estrogen levels were high than they did when levels were low. By contrast, the women were better on tasks involving spatial relationships when estrogen levels were low.

Even at their best, the Canadian researchers said at a symposium at the annual meeting of the Society for Neuroscience, the women did not perform as well as men do, on the average, with spatial tasks. But they added that even at their worst, the women as a group were better than men are on verbal tasks.

Dr. Kimura said men may also experience fluctuations in cognitive skills along with daily fluctuations in key male hormones. Testosterone is higher in the morning than the evening, she said, but no one has yet looked at how this might affect male thinking skills.

Dr. Blackman, chief of endocrinology at Johns Hopkins, says that there is a lot less information on men's brains than women's.

"We do know that men who have an endocrine disease and have abnormally low testosterone will improve on psychological function when they are given testosterone, but that is not the same as in older men with the so-called male menopause," Dr. Blackman notes. "They have lower testosterone, but if they are given supplemental testosterone, the effect will not be as dramatic as giving estrogen to women. Women lose ninety to ninety-five percent of their estrogen after menopause. Males lose thirty to fifty percent of their testosterone as they age. The magnitude of the deficit is different. We need some added insights before we can recommend testosterone replacement therapy in healthy middle-aged men as we recommend estrogen replacement therapy in postmenopausal women."[18]

ALZHEIMER'S AND DHEA

Alzheimer's patients have been found to have blood levels of DHEA 48 percent lower than their healthy peers.[19]

DHEA levels are close to the minimal at ages when the incidence of Alzheimer's disease begins to increase significantly, according to Dr. Eugene Roberts of the Department of Neurobiochemistry at the Beckman Research Institute, Duarte, California, and Dr. L. Jaime Fitten of the Department of Geropsychiatry, VA Medical Center, Sepulveda, California. The relative lack of significant circadian, monthly, seasonal, or annual rhythms in blood levels of DHEA suggests that its release may be buffered against large fluctuations, since it may be necessary for many important ongoing tissue functions, Drs. Roberts and Fitten say. In this light, its decrease in serum levels with age could presage changes in metabolism in many tissues that might have far-reaching consequences. Age-related progressive decrease in serum levels of

DHEA may reflect the gradual decreases in output of pituitary hormones. In one study, people 72–102 years had the same levels of adrenal hormones as individuals 35–62, but the levels of DHEA were significantly higher in the younger group and no stimulation by ACTH from the pituitary could increase DHEA levels. Thus, not only do the serum levels of DHEA fall with age in both sexes, but the ability to stimulate their release by ACTH from the adrenal gland, their chief source, is markedly reduced in the aging human.[20]

DHEA is now being administered to Alzheimer's patients in scientific studies. The French endocrinologist Etienne-Emile Baulieu is wagering that doses of DHEA will sharpen the mind even as they protect the body. The hormone helps brain cells grow in the lab, seems to improve rodents' short-term memory, and has even shown some effect in humans.[21]

"We've already seen some correlation between DHEA levels and mental acuity in older people," says Baulieu. People with Alzheimer's may have 58 percent less DHEA than matched controls of the same age. DHEA may be low in other degenerative diseases including diabetes and Parkinson's. DHEA deficiency should probably be treated in most cases. The body uses DHEA to produce male and female sex steroids such as testosterone and estrogen.

Kenneth Bonnet, M.D., of the Department of Psychiatry, New York University, and Richard P. Brown, Department of Psychiatry, Columbia University, reported on the effects of DHEA on memory in a forty-seven-year-old woman with a lifelong history of specific learning disabilities. She has complained of memory dysfunction and recurrent headaches for at least ten years. The patient was diagnosed variously as depressive and learning disabled by various professionals.

Her mother in middle age developed head tremor and Cushing's disease, which is related to overproduction of adrenal-gland hormones. Among the classic signs are a "moon" face, poor wound healing, and skin that is thin and fragile. The patient's brother was a high-functioning businessman, apparently normal but with mild head tremor similar to the mother's. The father had had a stroke in his late sixties while jogging and later developed moderate dementia due to multiple blood clots in the brain, with no other symptoms.

The forty-seven-year-old patient was found to have a low level of DHEA and was given DHEA replacement. Her memory was tested and an EEG (electroencephalogram) was taken to record her brain waves before and after DHEA replacement of 12.5 mg/kg per day. The tests showed that after her DHEA, her cognition was improved. The beneficial effects were most clear, the researchers said, in the EEG records, which are objective and not subjective.

The authors concluded that "replacement therapy of DHEA insufficiency has been applied for cognitive dysfunction largely in elderly populations showing gradual memory failure. In those individuals, evidence of DHEA insufficiency is indicative for replacement therapy." The case they presented, although a single-case study, indicates the advantages of testing younger individuals with complaints of persistent memory dysfunction or cognitive dysfunction that is not related to head trauma or tangible insult.

They emphasized that the patient benefited in cognitive enhancement but that some memory deficit remained unaltered in spite of DHEA replacement.

They said that DHEA should not be expected to overcome pathological memory dysfunction, but rather appears, in this case, to have enhanced the ability to attend to and to assimilate information.

The doctors said they were encouraged because the individual in the study had begun a self-sufficient business for the first time and maintained the benefit from modest dosage of oral DHEA.

HORMONES IN THE MOOD

A mood is an emotional state that may dominate your outlook and manner of expressing yourself for a time. Depression is a bad mood. It affects about 15 percent of the population, with the largest portion of the victims among the aging.

Stress of course can also cause a "bad mood," one of anxiety and irritability.

New research is showing that hormones involved in depression and stress can actually damage an area of the brain known as the hippocampus, a sea-horse-shaped structure in the brain vital for learning and memory and possessing many receptors for adrenal glucocorticoid (GC) hormones including hydrocortisone, epinephrine (adrenaline), and norepinephrine (noradrenaline), all of which pour out when we are under emotional stress.

Yvette I. Sheline, M.D., assistant professor of psychiatry at Washington University School of Medicine, St. Louis, found that women who have been clinically depressed have smaller hippocampi than women who have never suffered depressive episodes. Using high-resolution MRI (magnetic resonance imaging), Sheline's team also found that the more times a woman had been depressed, the smaller her brain's hippocampus was likely to be.[22]

Sheline says the data could mean that depressive episodes relate to one another, each event leaving "footprints" in the form of damaged nerve cells. Such damage may make a patient vulnerable to future bouts of depression, which would explain why depression recurs in some people months or years after they are treated.

Similar changes in the hippocampus were found in a recent

study of post–traumatic stress disorder patients. That study, from researchers at Yale, found that combat veterans had volume decreases in the hippocampus on the right side of the brain.[23] Because post–traumatic stress and depression involve similar chemical and hormonal changes, Sheline wondered whether she might find comparable damage in patients who had been clinically depressed.

When her team examined MRI scans in the depression study, they noted that while total brain size was comparable in the two groups of patients, the hippocampus was about 12 percent smaller in patients who had been depressed than in control subjects.

Is it the hormone cortisol released in large amounts in the brain during depressive episodes that causes the atrophy of the hippocampus, or are some people born with a smaller hippocampus, thus causing them to have recurrent bouts of depression?

Dr. Sheline says the only way to answer that chicken-and-egg question is to study patients under sixty. If a small hippocampus puts patients at risk, then depression could be observed at an early age. On the other hand, if depression is causing the hippocampus to shrink, there would be only minor differences in young subjects with large differences in older ones.

She says that animals studies support the latter hypothesis, and she is beginning studies to answer which comes first, the depression or the shrinking hippocampus.

The Stress Hormones and Your Brain

Stress may prematurely age the adult brain. National Institute on Aging grantee Philip Landfield, M.D., of the Bowman Gray School of Medicine, points out that the brain deterioration seen in older people and that seen in younger people with Cushing's syndrome, a rapid and premature form of aging associated with high levels of adrenal hormones, are quite similar. Over the years, Dr. Landfield has found that the blood levels of adrenal hormones in experimental animals correlate significantly with the degree of age-related changes in the brain.[24]

This seems quite logical when you consider that the brain structures that receive and send "emotional" information are called, collectively, the limbic system. One portion, about the size of a half-dollar, the amygdala, is involved in rage, anger, and fear behaviors. The nearby hippocampus is the target of the adrenal gland's stress hormones, which prepare the body for fight or flight. The continuous bombardment of stress hormones on the brain appears to kill off some of the stress hormone receptors in the hippocampus. As a result, researchers believe the hippocampus's ability to shut off the system weakens. Thus, through a feedback circuit, the brain's limbic system, the control center of emotions, gradually destroys itself.

Further proof of the effects stress hormone levels have on the brain in the aging has been found by researchers at Washington University, St. Louis. John Newcomer, M.D., assistant professor of psychiatry, gave a stress hormone to a number of volunteers, dexamethasone, to test declarative memory.

"Declarative memory can be thought of as 'shopping list' memory," says Dr. Newcomer. "It's the potentially conscious recall of facts and events over short intervals. The individuals in our study who received dexamethasone, in contrast to those given an inactive placebo, showed a decline in this particular kind of memory function."

Dr. Newcomer is interested in the effect of stress hormones in the hippocampus, the structure involved in declarative memory. Prior to the study, there was a variety of evidence from animal models and cultured cells that glucocorticoids (of which dexamethasone is one) might impair the function of hippocampal nerve cells, so before his experiment, he had the idea that glucocorticoid treatment would affect memory.

"The data confirms the hypothesis. We knew stress hormones

had an effect on cell function. Now we know, at least in part, how that cellular effect translates into a functional effect in the human brain," Dr. Newcomer concludes.[25]

Can Hormones Help?

While scientists are striving to understand the physical effects on the brain of mood, no one doubts that hormones affect moods and that supplemental hormones may change moods.

If hormone replacement therapy can put a woman more in the mood for sex, can it elevate her mood in general? Menopausal witches have long been part of the legend of menopause. "The change of life" is associated with aging and illness and often seen as a medical condition rather than a normal transition. These negative perceptions color information dissemination and decision making by women and their health care providers. To address these problems, researchers such as those in Pittsburgh looked at three different groups of women:

- Menstruating
- Menopausal with no treatment
- Menopausal on hormone therapy

The study showed that menopausal women suffered no more anxiety, depression, anger, nervousness, or feelings of stress than the group of menstruating women in the same age range.[26] In addition, although more hot flashes were reported by the menopausal women not taking hormones, surprisingly they had better overall mental health than the other two groups. The women taking hormones worried more about their bodies and were somewhat more depressed. However, this could be caused by the hormones themselves. It's also possible that women who voluntarily take hormones tend to be more conscious of their bodies in the first place. The researchers caution that their study includes only healthy women, so results may apply only to them. Other studies show that women already taking hormones who are experiencing mood or behavioral problems sometimes respond well to a change in dosage or type of estrogen.

The Pittsburgh findings are supported by a New England Research Institute study that found menopausal women were no more depressed than the general population: about 10 percent are occasionally depressed and 5 percent are persistently depressed. The exception is women who undergo surgical menopause. Their depression rate is reportedly double that of women who have had a natural menopause.[27]

It is difficult to separate out the biological from the social reasons why some women have a traumatic menopause experience. The hands of the biological clock strike usually just as their children are grown and leaving home, and their husbands are at the apex of their careers. Many women feel that with their reproduction function finished, they are old and useless.

On the other hand, the uncomfortable symptoms of hormonal changes may affect mood. Geriatrician Dr. Howard Fillit points out that while no major depression is associated with menopause, there are subclinical (not obvious by usual medical tests) complaints of

- Irritability
- Difficulty in concentrating
- Memory

"If you are up all night with flushes and may have a dysfunctional sex life, sleep disorders, no wonder you are irritable," he says.

Dr. Fillit points out that there are estrogen receptors in the hippocampus and the amygdala, both areas involved in memory and learning, not just in sexual behavior. Estrogen receptors are in specific parts of the brain, and estrogen has a direct effect on nerve growth factors.

He says studies have shown that estrogen replacement affects higher cognitive functions. "Studies have shown estrogen acts as a monoamine oxidase inhibitor [MAOI]," he notes.

Monoamine oxidase is an enzyme in the brain that is linked to depression and which some antidepressant pharmaceuticals inhibit.

Testosterone and Mood

The male hormones may have a wide range of adverse psychiatric and behavioral effects.[28] Much is unknown about the effects of anabolic-androgenic steroids on libido in men and in women, and how they are different. Anabolic-androgenic steroids may both relieve and cause depression, for example. Cessation or diminished use of male hormones may result in depression. Testosterone has been widely reported to be associated with aggression, particularly in response to provocation.

In elderly men with low levels of male hormone, preliminary studies have shown that testosterone replacement not only improves libido but also significantly increases musculoskeletal mass and strength. However, adverse effects have included increases in hematocrit and prostate specific antigen.[29]

In women, it reportedly does the same. Dr. B. B. Sherwin of the Department of Psychology, McGill University, Montreal, Canada, concludes that testosterone is the hormone "most critically implicated in the maintenance of libido, or sexual desire, in women just as it is in men."[30]

DHEA and Mood

DHEA is found in equal concentrations in the brain and the adrenal gland, which plays a part in the stress reaction, as pointed out earlier.

Dr. William Regelson and his colleagues Dr. Mohammed Kalimi and Roger Loria, from the Medical College of Virginia, say studies at 90 mg per day showed improvement in mood and energy in one-third of the patients in a nonrandomized study. This effect might relate to the high testosterone levels resulting from DHEA metabolism, as they saw hirsutism and increased libido in several of the female patients.[31]

This elevation in mood is not surprising in view of DHEA-S marketing in Europe alone or combined with estrogen or post-menopausal depression.

The Virginia researchers said that Italian researchers have studied DHEA in depression or fatigue syndromes with significant clinical results.

Pregnenolone—Another Brain Hormone Tool

Pregnenolone is a steroid hormone produced by the adrenal gland and manufactured from cholesterol. It is also produced in the brain and nerves. As with other hormones, pregnenolone levels decrease with age. It was used to treat arthritis in the past but was pretty much abandoned with the more powerful anti-inflammatory steroids. Recently, it has aroused interest as a neurohormone. It improves transmission, communication, between nerve cells and is believed to have an effect on memory. Pregnenolone is made in the supporting tissue cells of the brain and can both stimulate and calm the brain. As a so-called excitatory neurohormone, it activates the neuroreceptors that take up glutamate. On the other hand, it seems able to calm the brain by activating gamma aminobutyric acid (GABA) receptors—the same receptors that receive Valium.[32] It can also reportedly rehabilitate spinal cord injury.[33]

Researchers at the University of St. Louis are about to begin a study of pregnenolone and memory in older humans. They have already done a study in animals that showed the hormone was low

212 THE ANTI-AGING HORMONES

in older mice with learning and memory deficits. Administration of the hormone after training improved the animal's retention of what they had learned.[34]

Melatonin and Mood

Melatonin, as described in chapter 6, is intimately tied to our biological clock and to sleep. Can it also have an effect on our moods? To determine if the hormone had any behavioral effects, researchers at the Massachusetts Institute of Technology (MIT) gave pharmacologic doses to fourteen healthy men. Melatonin significantly decreased self-reported alertness and increased sleepiness as measured by the Profile of Mood States and the Stanford Sleepiness Scale on self-report mood questionnaires. The effects were brief. Melatonin also affected performance, slowing choice-reaction time but concurrently decreasing errors of commission. Fine motor performance was not impaired, nor were memory and visual sensitivity on administered tests.[39]

The MIT researchers concluded that melatonin administered orally in pharmacological quantities has significant but short-acting sedative-like properties.

Output of the pineal gland is also abnormal in the depressed. Emerging findings suggest that investigation of pineal function and its melatonin hormone may be of use in monitoring antidepressant effects, in diagnosis of manic depression, and in investigation of a variety of rhythm disorders, including seasonal affective disorder, jet lag, and shift work.[40]

The Brain, Hormones, and Depression

There are multiple abnormalities in growth hormone regulation in the depressed. Identifying its participation in depression is difficult because growth hormone response is susceptible to change, depending on age, sex, menstrual-cycle phase, menstrual status, stress, and other factors. So, as of now, it is not a practical diagnostic tool.[41]

Approximately 25 percent of depressed patients have changes in their thyrotropin-releasing hormone from an area of the brain called the hypothalamus, which in turn stimulates the pituitary gland to release its hormone, which in turn causes the thyroid gland to release its hormone. Thyroid hormone controls the rates of chemical reactions in the body. Generally, the more thyroid hormone the faster the body works. This test has limited clinical use because similar abnormalities are seen in alcoholism and can be produced by starvation.[42] Thyrotropin is also believed by some researchers to play a part in memory function.

Self-Made Tranquilizers and Stimulants

What happens to neurohormones as we age? Neurohormones are chemical messengers sent by nerves from one to another. So far, more than fifty have been identified, and they fit into several basic families with the "last name" *ergic,* which means *energy.* They include the *cholinergic,* which has acetylcholine, vital to memory; *adrenergic,* with epinephrine and norepinephrine, stimulators from the adrenal gland; the *dopaminergic,* with dopamine, vital to movement; *GABA-ergic* with the inhibitor GABA; and *serotoninergic,* with its mood elevator serotonin. There are many other neurohormones, some known and some yet to be discovered. The neurohormones cause either excitement or inhibition. That they even exist has been known only for a relatively short time.

Neurohormones are generally referred to as *endorphins* and, like the more recognized hormones, have effects far from their site of origin. Endorphins are similar to heroin in their composition and operation. They prevent pain and invoke a feeling of euphoria. The difference is that they are many times more powerful and are manufactured by our bodies for our own use.[43] Opiates such as heroin cause an effect that can last for a long time, while endorphins are released as a temporary reaction to stress. The neurohormones are what keep us from feeling immediate pain during stress from a traumatic injury during a sporting event or an accident. And like opiates manufactured outside the body, endorphins in the body can be somewhat addictive. Runner's high, that feeling of euphoria that keeps the athlete going, is believed to be due, in large part, to the release of endorphins due to the physical stress. Enjoyment of music, too, is said to produce the release of endorphins.[44]

A number of pharmaceutical firms and university scientists are trying to develop medications that will prevent the destruction or increase the amount of acetylcholine in the brains of the aging, since this hormone is believed to be a key factor in the development of memory loss, including the devastating type that is characteristic of Alzheimer's disease.

The medication levodopa is used to treat Parkinson's disease, in which movement disorders are caused by a gradual deterioration in certain nerve centers inside the brain. Levodopa, a precursor of dopamine, is able to cross the natural blood-brain barrier, where it is believed to be converted to dopamine in the brains of Parkinson's suffers, who are usually over forty years old.

Endorphins are known to play a part in pain, and indeed, the levels of endorphins found in both the blood and joint fluids of people suffering from rheumatoid arthritis, gout, and similar diseases were considerably lower than levels in persons without these conditions.

Endorphin research really got under way in the 1980s. Some neuroscientists are devoting their whole careers to studying just one neurohormone. Much is yet to be discovered about how aging affects neurohormones and vice versa. Medications are already on the market or about to enter the market that will treat many of the ills associated with aging with synthetic versions of these extremely powerful self-made chemicals that play such a large part in our physical and emotional well-being.

Minding Your Hormones

Most scientists agree that emotions are different from rational thought, perception through the senses, and memory function, yet emotions interplay with all three. As we grow older and are exposed to the highs and lows of life, our emotions may become harder to control. Our moods may become more depressed. The hormones that are released from the brain and the endocrine glands not only respond to emotions, they may cause them. John Locke, the English philosopher, observed, "A sound mind in a sound body is a short but full description of a happy state in this world." As scientists learn more about how hormones act from and on the brain, protection against memory loss and depression will more effectively help to keep the mind sound.

10. Anti-Aging Hormone Research and Your More Youthful Future

Are we programmed to live only to a certain age?

When I was a young newspaper reporter, my editors assigned me to write about golden wedding anniversaries because they were a rare phenomenon. Today, they are unremarkable, and seventy-fifth wedding anniversaries are not that unusual. The obituary columns today also have more and more stories about people departing this earth after 100 to 110 years. In the present, the sixty-five-year-old is considered the youth of old age.

Living long is really not the objective of most people. Living well for many years is.

One main feature of aging is the progressive loss of coordination between many different rhythmic—circadian and seasonal—functions of the body, resulting in maladaptation to environmental factors such as light, temperature, stress, and germs. Common patterns of aging are, in fact, sleep-cycle alterations, temperature defects, depression, decreased immunity, heart problems, and cancer.[1] There is no doubt, therefore, that many aspects of so-called *metabolic* aging depend upon a profound derangement of the endocrine gland products known as hormones.

Until recently, according to Dr. S. Michael Jazwinski of the department of biochemistry and molecular biology, Louisiana State University Medical School, New Orleans, biogerontology was a backwater of biology, but progress in the qualitative and quantitative analysis of longevity has led to its revolution in aging research. This research has revealed that extended longevity is frequently associated with an enhanced metabolic capacity and response to stress.[2]

The phenomenon known as menopause is now recognized as having more impact than just closing the door on fertility. It is acknowledged to affect urinary continence, nutrient absorption and metabolism, bone and mineral metabolism, blood pressure and cardiovascular function, memory and cognition, daily rhythms, and the progression of age-related diseases.[3] The evidence that both the ovary and the brain are key pacemakers in menopause is now pretty well established. And because it occurs now, on the average, in the middle of the life span, researchers believe it is an excellent model for studying what actually happens to the human body during aging.

Dr. Marc Blackman, Chief of the Division of Endocrinology at Johns Hopkins–Bayview Medical Center and director of one of the biggest and most exciting hormone-intervention-in-aging projects funded by the National Institute on Aging, is himself a member of the baby boomer generation just reaching the fifth decade of life.

"I'm trying to be dispassionate," he said, laughing, "but there is very exciting research going on worldwide with the hormone system because it is so closely related to aging."

But, Dr. Blackman urges caution: "It is very early in the research. We have to first prove these interventions are safe and effective. The population is aging and we have to understand the aging process better. The endocrine, immune, and nervous systems are very complicated. They are way stations with information going each way, and there are all sorts of different combinations. This is intriguing in the scientific sense."

He says that the implications are that once we understand more about aging, we will be able to prevent, rather than repair, some of the disabilities that are now associated with aging.

He said the work with estrogen and Alzheimer's is an example. But, he said, just because melatonin and DHEA are available over the counter does not mean they are completely safe and effective.

Dr. Blackman notes, "We don't know enough about them yet. There is reason to believe that these hormones and the others, such as growth hormone and testosterone, all of these manifest age-dependent decreases. All of them contribute separately and in combination to some of the changes that occur in aging, and there are compelling reasons to study them both separately and interactively. There needs to be careful research. These studies have to be done with active compounds and placebos in a controlled manner."

He said the results of the current studies and the therapeutic use of various hormones in normal aging is not that far away—perhaps two to five years. And while that may seem a long time for those anxious to have a vigorous old age, it is quick as scientific research goes.

Dr. Blackman said that while there are promising results with hormones, general physicians should not rush into prescribing them and people should not insist on taking them until efficacy and safety are proven. Hormones are powerful.

"Too little or too much of a hormone is wrong," he says, and we have to be sure of efficacy and safety.

Fran Kaiser, M.D., professor of medicine at the University of St. Louis, Missouri, and one of the prime hormone researchers, says of hormone replacement therapy:

"No one size fits all! You have to weigh the benefits against the risks, for you as an individual. If the benefits outweigh the risks, then hormone replacement therapy is for you. If they don't, it isn't."

Today, however, Dr. Blackman and the other scientists quoted in his book agree that there is more hope than ever before that we can be healthy and vigorous into a very old chronological age. Thanks to the increasing body of knowledge about our hormones and their function and scientists' ability to diagnose and provide therapeutic replacement, many are already benefiting. We are just at the beginning of hormonal intervention in aging.

It is feasible right now for you to walk into a doctor's office, have an analysis of your hormone levels, and have them supplemented if they are low. It may be possible, as you read in chapters 3 and 4, to use growth factors to rebuild damaged or missing tissue. Immunity may be restored, and skin, bones, and muscles may be rebuilt, with hormone therapy. Peaceful sleep and a happy sex life may be possible even in the ninth and tenth decades of life.

Not only will we be able soon to greatly extend life, we will be able to repair defects and to banish pain and suffering—be it diabetes, heart trouble, cancer, or whatever.

Millions and millions of healthy aged will want to continue to live life to the fullest. We will come to know hundred-year marriages, families of at least six generations, and living experiences and knowledge of centuries' vintage.

If hormones and other age-affecting chemicals are fully understood, we will be able to maintain a physical and mental condition of a generation or more younger. We will not develop the age-connected diseases that are today overburdening doctors and health care facilities. And we will be better able to withstand environmental stress.

But, as pointed out in this book a number of times, such therapies are always a part of a Faustian bargain. No effective chemical therapy is without potential side effects. It is unwise for you to take therapeutic doses of hormones without knowing the benefits versus the risks.

Arm yourself with knowledge. Make use of those hormone therapies that will be beneficial to you, then decide how you are going to fulfill yourself in a healthy, long life.

The Rand Corporation, which specializes in anticipating breakthroughs in various aspects of technology and science, predicted in the early 1970s that chemical control of aging would be available by the year 2025, with artificial organs made of plastic and electronic components available by 1990. Biochemicals to stimulate the growth of new organs and limbs were predicted by 2020. As you have read in this book, we are ahead of those predictions.

The always conservative American Medical Association's Council on Medical Services said at the same time that with intelligent application of existing knowledge, we should all live past ninety, and many beyond one hundred.

How long is the ultimate human life span? It could be as varied as the life span between species and among the same species. Some plants are annuals and do not survive the first winter, while the giant sequoia tree lives 3,000 years and the bristlecone pine 4,600 years. The dog, who suffers all the same ills as we humans, including heart disease, diabetes, and cancer, lives twelve to eighteen years. The species closest to us physiologically, the chimpanzee, lives from thirty to forty years. Some gerontologists opt for about one hundred twenty years as the ultimate human life span. Others are convinced it is infinite.

The English author Jonathan Swift really summed it up when he said, "Every man desires to live long, but no man would be old."

As we enter the twenty-first century, most of us will live twice as long as those who lived at the turn of the twentieth century. Gerontologists are making tremendous strides as demonstrated by the many exciting research results described in this book. Chances are excellent that you will have the time and the vigor to learn about your world within and without. You will then know the reality of Robert Browning's "Grow old along with me! The best is yet to be."

ACETYLCHOLINE. A neurotransmitter that is released by nerve cells and acts on either other nerve cells or on muscles and organs throughout the body. It plays an important role in learning and memory.

ACTH. Abbreviation for adrenocorticotropic hormone (*see*), a hormone controller.

ACTIVE IMMUNITY. Immunity produced by the body in response to stimulation by a disease-causing organism or a vaccine.

ADDISON'S DISEASE. A progressive disorder resulting from shrinkage of the adrenal gland and the subsequent decrease in the amount of hormones produced by this gland. Early symptoms include weakness and fatigue. Later, brown spots appear on the skin because of hyperpigmentation. Weight loss, low blood pressure, nausea, and diarrhea also occur. Pres. John Kennedy suffered from this disorder.

ADRENAL GLAND. About the size of grapes, the two adrenal glands lie on top of each of the kidneys. Each adrenal gland has two parts. The first part is the medulla, which produces epinephrine and norepinephrine, two hormones that play a part in controlling heart rate and blood pressure. Signals from the brain stimulate production of these hormones. The second part is the adrenal cortex, which produces three groups of steroid hormones. The hormones in one group control the levels of various chemicals in the body. For example, they prevent the loss of too much sodium and water into the urine. Aldosterone is the most important hormone in this group. The hormones in the second group have a number of functions. One is to help convert carbohydrates, or starches, into energy-providing glycogen in the liver. Hydrocortisone is the main hormone in this group. The third group consists of the male hormone androgen and the female hormones estrogen and progesterone.

ADRENOCORTICOTROPIC HORMONE. ACTH. Stimulates the outer layer of the adrenal gland (*see*) and is used as an anti-inflammatory medication.

AGONIST. A hormone, drug, or neurotransmitter that triggers a response like a natural substance by occupying the cell receptor site usually reserved for that substance.

AIDS. Acquired immunodeficiency syndrome. A life-threatening disease caused by a virus and characterized by a breakdown of the body's immune system.

ALZHEIMER'S DISEASE. A deterioration of the brain with severe memory impairment.

AMINO ACIDS. Building blocks of proteins. There are twenty common amino acids: alanine, arginine, asparagine, aspartic acid, cysteine, glutamic acid, glutamine, glycine, histidine, isoleucine, leucine, lysine, methionine, phenylalanine, proline, serine, threonine, tryptophan, tyrosine, and valine.

ANABOLIC. Drugs related to male hormones, sometimes given for "upbuilding" action, to stimulate growth, weight gain, strength, and appetite. They are being studied to counteract some of the weight and muscle loss in the aged.

ANALOG. A compound similar in structure but not identical in composition.

ANDROGEN. Male hormones produced in the body for normal sexual development. Natural and synthetic androgens are used to replace natural hormones when the body is unable to produce enough on its own, to stimulate the beginning of puberty in boys and to treat certain types of breast cancer in women. Now being studied intensively for their use in counteracting some of the dysfunctions caused during aging.

ANDROGENIC. Producing masculine characteristics.

ANGIOGENESIS GROWTH FACTOR (AGF). Plays a part in the growth of blood vessels.

ANTAGONIST. A substance, such as a hormone, drug, or enzyme inhibitor, that diminishes or prevents the action of another substance in the body.

ANTERIOR. The front of a structure.

ANTIBODY. A protein in the blood formed to neutralize or destroy foreign substances or organisms (antigens). Each antibody is tailor-made for an antigen.

ANTICHOLINERGIC. The blocking of acetylcholine receptors, which results in the inhibition of nerve-impulse transmission.

ANTIESTROGEN. Any substance that prevents the full biological effects of estrogen (*see*) on responsive tissues, either by producing antagonistic effects on the target tissue or by blocking the effects of estrogen.

ANTIGEN. A foreign protein that can cause an immune response by stimulating the production of antibodies in the body.

ANTIOXIDANTS. Compounds that neutralize oxygen radicals. Some are enzymes while others are nutrients and reportedly hormones. High levels of antioxidants have been associated with healthier and longer life spans.

APOE-4. One form of the apoE gene, which produces a protein found in the brains in people with Alzheimer's disease more than in the general population. The other two forms of the gene, apoE-2 and apoE-3, may protect against the disease.

APOLIPOPROTEIN E. A protein that carries cholesterol in the blood and that appears to play some role in the brain.

ARTERIOSCLEROSIS. Also called hardening of the arteries, this includes a number of conditions that cause artery walls to thicken and lose elasticity.

ARTERY. Any one of a series of blood vessels that carry blood from the heart to various parts of the body. Arteries have thick, elastic walls that can thicken and lose elasticity.

ATHEROSCLEROSIS. A form of arteriosclerosis in which the artery walls become thick and irregular due to deposits of fat, cholesterol, and other substances. The buildup is sometimes called plaque. As the walls become obstructed, blood flow is reduced or stopped.

AUTOIMMUNE DISEASE. A disease, such as rheumatoid arthritis or lupus, in which the body manufactures antibodies against its own tissues and damages itself.

AUTONOMIC NERVOUS SYSTEM. The division of the nervous system that regulates the involuntary vital functions, such as the activity of the heart and breathing. Governs the excitation and relaxation of muscles. One part of the system, the sympathetic, widens airways to the lungs and increases the flow of blood to the arms and legs and prepares the body for fight or flight. The other part, the parasympathetic, slows the heart rate and stimulates the flow of digestive juices. Although the sympathetic and parasympathetic cooperate in the functional rhythm of most organs, the muscles surrounding the blood vessels are affected only by the signals from the sympathetic system. The trigger for constriction or relaxation of the blood vessels involves two sets of receptors, the alpha and beta. Among the compounds that act on the sympathetic nervous system are epinephrine and norepinephrine (*see both*). Among the compounds that act on the parasympathetic system is acetylcholine (*see*).

AXON. The tubelike part of a neuron that transmits outgoing signals to other cells.

B CELL. White blood cells that are processed or derived from bone marrow and play an important part in immunity. Also called B lymphocytes.

BETA-BLOCKERS. Drugs that slow heart activity and thus lower blood pressure. They are used to treat angina (chest pain), high blood pressure, and irregular heart rhythms. They are given after a heart attack to reduce the likelihood of fatal irregular heartbeats or further damage to the heart muscle. These drugs are also prescribed to improve heart function in damaged hearts. Beta-blockers may also be used to prevent migraine headaches, to reduce anxiety, to control fluid pressure in the eye, and for an overactive thyroid. There are two types of beta receptors. Beta 1 receptors are located mainly in the heart muscle, and beta 2 are in the airways and blood vessels. Beta-blockers work by occupying the beta receptors in these areas, thus blocking the stimulating action of the nerve-stimulating chemical norepinephrine. Thus they reduce the force and speed of the heartbeat, prevent the dilation of the airways to the lungs, and prevent the dilation of the blood vessels surrounding the brain and leading to the extremities. Drugs for the heart act mainly on beta 1 receptors. Beta-blockers are usually not prescribed for people who have poor circulation, particularly in the legs and arms. Beta-blockers should not be stopped suddenly after prolonged use because it may worsen the symptoms of the disorders for which they were prescribed. They should not be taken with foods, beverages, or over-the-counter medications that contain caffeine or alcohol or are high in sodium. The combination may increase heart rate or elevate blood pressure.

BIOCHEMICAL. A substance that is produced by a chemical reaction in a living organism. Some can also be made in the laboratory.

BIOTECHNOLOGY. The scientific manipulation by genetic engineering and other cutting-edge biomedical endeavors of living organisms or compounds of living organisms to produce useful products to improve human health, industrial efficiency, and food production.

BLOOD-BRAIN BARRIER. Some natural body substances, drugs, and chemicals circulating in the blood are unable to reach active brain cells because of the blood-brain barrier. The mechanism, including tightly packed cells and chemicals, serves as a selective traffic officer that permits some substances to "go" and others to be blocked. It is believed to be a natural protective mechanism against substances that might harm the brain.

BONE MARROW. Soft tissue located in the cavities of the bones. Responsible for producing blood cells.

CALORIE. A unit of heat used in measuring body metabolism and the fattening propensities of foods.

CARBOHYDRATE. Starches and sugars contain a high proportion of carbohydrates. These are chemicals that contain carbon, hydrogen, and oxygen. Gums and mucilages are complex carbohydrates and are ingredients in soothing herbs and medications.

CARCINOGEN. A substance that causes cancer.

CARCINOGENESIS. The development of cancer.

CARPAL TUNNEL SYNDROME. Pertaining to compression of a large nerve that passes from the wrist to the hand causing tingling and numbness of the fingers.

CELL. The smallest living unit that is able to grow and reproduce. A single cell may be a complete organism such as a bacterium or may be a specialized unit that is part of a large plant or animal.

CEREBRAL CORTEX. The part of the brain most involved in learning, language, and reasoning.

CHOLESTEROL. A waxy substance resembling fat in its properties, closely related to the sex hormones and vitamin D. It is present in brain tissue, bile, nerve sheaths, and all tissues.

CHOLINERGIC NEURONS. Nerve cells that contain acetylcholine and those that are stimulated by it. These nerves are involved in memory.

CHOLINESTERASE. The enzyme that processes the neurotransmitter acetylcholine. There is a great deal of scientific interest in this enzyme, particularly in the study of Alzheimer's disease, because it is believed to be involved in poor memory function.

CHRONOPHARMACOLOGY. The timing of medications so they are administered when they are most effective.

CIRCADIAN RHYTHM. Internal biological rhythm that cycles around twenty-four hours.

CLINICAL TRIALS, PHASES I, II, AND III. See PHASE I, II, and III.

COGNITIVE FUNCTIONS. All aspects of thinking, perceiving, and remembering.

COLLAGEN. Fibers of connective tissue that support the body.

COMPLEMENT. A complex series of blood proteins whose action "complements" the work of antibodies (*see*). Complement destroys bacteria, produces inflammation, and regulates immune reactions.

CONTROLS. In an experiment, the reference base with which the results are compared. In experiments with patients, it usually means subjects matched for age, gender, and physical condition are divided into groups in which some receive the active medication and/or routine and others receive a placebo (*see*) while undergoing the same routine. The results are then compared to determine if the active medication was effective.

CORONARY ARTERY DISEASE. Disease of the heart caused by atherosclerotic narrowing of the coronary arteries; likely to produce chest pain (angina pectoris) or heart attack.

CORTEX. The surface layer of an organ such as the brain or adrenal gland. The cortex of an organ has different functions from its inner part; for example, the adrenal cortex produces hormones entirely different from those of its inner part.

CORTICOSTEROIDS. Substances secreted by the cortex of the adrenal gland having the properties of hormones. Cortisone, hydrocortisone, prednisone, and many other corticosteroids are used in medicine.

CORTICOTROPIN-RELEASING FACTOR (CRF). A neurotransmitter involved in appetite and stress reactions.

CRUCIFEROUS VEGETABLES. A family of plants characterized by flowers and fruits that bear a cross. The genus being studied intensively for their health benefits are the *Brassica,* which include brussels sprouts, cauliflower, and broccoli. These vegetables contain quantities of some substances that have been shown to inhibit chemically induced cancers in animals.

CYTOKINES. Naturally occurring proteins that regulate or modify the growth of specific cells.

DEMENTIA. A condition in which cognitive functions decline.

DENDRITES. Spiderlike projections from the cell body that receive and send messages between nerve cells.

DHEA. Dehydroepiandrosterone. Produced in the adrenal glands, it is a weak male hormone and a precursor to some other hormones, including testosterone and estrogen.

DIFFERENTIATION. The biochemical and structural changes by which cells become specialized in form and function. Why one cell becomes a skin cell and another a brain cell.

DNA. Deoxyribonucleic acid. A large molecule that carries the genetic information necessary for all cellular functions. The DNA molecule consists of four bases—adenine, cytosine, guanidine, and thymine—and a sugar-phosphate backbone, arranged in two connected strands. Damage to DNA and the rate at which this damage is repaired may help determine the rate of aging.

DOPAMINE. Dopamine is a neurotransmitter (*see*) involved in movement and mood. It is an intermediate in tyrosine metabolism and the precursor of norepinephrine and epinephrine.

DOUBLE-BLIND CLINICAL TRIAL. A placebo (*see*) is designed to look, feel, and taste exactly like the substance being tested, so that neither the investigator nor the subjects know who is taking the active ingredient.

EEG. Electroencephalogram; a brain-wave tracing or record.

EKG. Electrocardiogram, which records contraction of the heart muscle.

ENDOCRINE GLANDS. Specialized glands in the body that adjust the activities of the body to the changing demands of the external and internal environment. They secrete hormones directly into the bloodstream to affect other organs at a distance.

ENDOMETRIUM. The tissue lining the uterus.

ENDORPHINS. Self-made tranquilizers and painkillers. Each endorphin is composed of a chain of amino acids and acts on the nervous system to reduce pain.

ENKEPHALINS. Self-made painkillers including endorphins.

ENZYME. A complex chemical, a protein, produced by living cells, that promotes the chemical processes of life without itself being altered.

EPIDERMIS. The outer portion of the skin.

EPINEPHRINE. Adrenaline. The major hormone of the adrenal gland, epinephrine increases heart rate and contractions, constricts or dilates blood vessels, relaxes the muscles in the lungs and smooth muscles in the intestines, and helps process sugar and fat.

EPITHELIAL TISSUES. See EPITHELIUM.

EPITHELIUM. The cellular covering of internal and external body surfaces, including the lining of vessels and small cavities. The epithelium consists of cells joined by small amounts of cementing substances and is classified according to the number of layers and shape of the cells.

ERT. Estrogen replacement therapy (*see*).

ERYTHROPOIESIS. Red blood cell development.

ESTROGEN. A hormone produced by the ovaries, it is mainly responsible for female sexual characteristics. Estrogen influences bone mass by slowing or halting bone loss, improving retention of calcium by the kidneys, and improving the absorption of dietary calcium by the intestines. Estrogen is given to relieve menopausal symptoms, prevent or relieve aging changes in the vagina and urethra, and to help prevent osteoporosis (*see*). Potential adverse reactions include increased risk of uterine cancer, increased frequency of gallstones, accelerated growth of preexisting fibroid tumors of the uterus, fluid retention, nausea, rash, hives, itching, headache, nervous tension, irritability, accentuation of migraine, bloating, diarrhea, pigmentation of the face, postmenopausal bleeding, deep-vein blood clots (less likely with conjugated estrogens), increased blood pressure, and decreased sugar tolerance. May cause swelling and tenderness of breasts, milk production, and increased vaginal secretions. When taking estrogens, it is recommended that salt be used sparingly if fluid retention is a problem. Smoking cigarettes may increase the side effects of estrogen.

ESTROGEN REPLACEMENT THERAPY (ERT). A treatment that restores estrogen when natural estrogen production in the ovaries is dramatically reduced due to the onset of menopause. Physicians question if ERT increases the risk of breast cancer, especially for women who have a family history of breast cancer. See ESTROGEN.

EXPEDITED PROCESS. Under a plan implemented by the FDA early in 1989, Phases II and III of clinical trials may be combined to shave two to three years from the development process for those medicines that show sufficient promise in early testing and are targeted against serious and life-threatening diseases such as AIDS and cancer. Approval time for these drugs in 1994 averaged 5.9 months. See also PHASES I, II, and III, and FDA APPROVAL.

FATTY ACIDS. Compounds of carbon, hydrogen, and oxygen that combine with glycerol to make fats.

FDA APPROVAL. Once the FDA approves a new drug application (NDA) (*see*) the new medicine may be prescribed by all physicians. The company that produces the new drug is required to continue to submit periodic reports to the FDA, including any cases of adverse reactions and appropriate quality-control records. For some medicines, the FDA requires additional studies to evaluate long-term effects.

FIBRIN. An insoluble protein formed in blood as its clots. Derived from fibrinogen.

FIBRINOGEN. A clotting factor; an inactive plasma protein that is activated by thrombin to form fibrin (*see*).

FOLLICLE-STIMULATING HORMONE (FSH). A hormone from the front part of the pituitary gland that controls the maturation and function of the ovaries and testes.

FREE RADICALS. Molecules with unpaired electrons that react readily with other molecules. Oxygen free radicals, produced during metabolism, damage cells and may be responsible for aging in tissues and organs.

FSH. Follicle-stimulating hormone (*see*).

GABA. Gamma-aminobutyric acid (*see*).

GAMMA-AMINOBUTYRIC ACID (GABA). A compound found in high concentrations in the brain, it functions as an inhibitory chemical messenger.

GENE. The smallest genetic unit of a chromosome. It is a piece of DNA that contains the hereditary information for the production of a specific protein.

GENE THERAPY. The replacement of a defective gene in an organism suffering from a genetic disease.

GENETIC ENGINEERING. The technique of removing, modifying, or adding genetic material in living cells to produce a new substance or new function. This includes adding or deleting genes, as well as preventing, or turning off, the expression of particular genes.

GERONTOLOGISTS. Doctors who study aging.

GF. Growth factors (*see*).

GH. Human growth hormone (*see*).

GHRH. Growth hormone–releasing hormone (*see*).

GLAND. A cell or organ that makes and releases hormones or other substances used in the body. *Endocrine* glands secrete their products, hormones, into the bloodstream; *exocrine* glands, such as sweat glands, secrete to body surfaces or elsewhere, via ducts or channels.

GLUCAGON. A neurotransmitter (*see*) that is involved in sugar metabolism and hunger.

GLUCOSE. Sugar that occurs naturally in blood, grape, and corn sugars. A source of energy for animals and plants. Sweeter than sucrose. It is used medicinally for nutritional purposes and for diabetic coma. Used to soothe the skin.

GLUCOSE TOLERANCE. The ability to properly metabolize sugar.

GLUCOSE TOLERANCE TEST. A test for early diabetes and other metabolic disorders. It measures a patient's ability to reduce blood sugar levels at a normal rate. After fasting, a blood sugar level is taken as a baseline and the person is given a measured amount of dissolved sugar to drink. Blood sugar levels are then taken periodically. Abnormal rise or persistence of blood sugar is indicative of diabetes.

GONADS. The primary sex glands, ovaries and testes.

GROWTH FACTORS. Like hormones, growth factors trigger a variety of bodily functions. The body's own growth factors are produced by almost all tissues. Some regulate normal processes, such as maintaining blood supply, while others come into play when things go awry during illness.

GROWTH HORMONE. Somatotropin. A protein produced by the pituitary gland that is involved in cell growth.

GROWTH HORMONE–RELEASING HORMONE (GHRH). A hormone from the hypothalamus (*see*) that triggers the pituitary gland to secrete hGH. Researchers have synthesized it and are using it in an effort to boost growth hormone.

HDL. High-density lipoprotein cholesterol, the "good" cholesterol thought to have a cleansing effect in the bloodstream.

HELPER T CELLS. A subset of T cells that are essential for turning on antibody production, activating killer T cells, and initiating many other immune responses.

HEMOGLOBIN. The coloring matter of red blood cells that carries oxygen.

HEPARIN-BINDING GROWTH FACTOR (HBGF). It is involved in the growth of blood vessels and smooth-muscle cells and may be important in tumor growth, wound healing, and the development of fat-blocked arteries.

HERPES VARICELLA ZOSTER. Shingles. Painful blisters on the skin that follow nerve pathways. It may appear in adulthood as a result of having had chicken pox as a child.

hGH. Human growth hormone (*see*).

HIPPOCAMPUS. A structure deep within the brain involved in memory storage.

HIV. Human immunodeficiency virus, which causes AIDS.

HORMONE REPLACEMENT THERAPY (HRT). The use of estrogen combined with progestin for the treatment of menopausal symptoms and the prevention of some long-term effects of menopause.

HRT. Hormone replacement therapy (*see*).

HUMAN GROWTH HORMONE (hGH). A product of the pituitary gland that appears to play a role in body composition and muscle and bone strength. It is released through the action of another growth factor, growth hormone–releasing hormone, which is produced in the brain. It works by stimulating production of insulin-like growth factor, which comes mainly from the liver. All three are being studied for their potential to strengthen muscle and bones and prevent frailty among older people.

HUMORAL IMMUNITY. Immune protection provided by soluble factors such as antibodies, which circulate in the body's fluids or "humors," primarily serum and lymph.

HYBRIDOMA. The cell produced by fusing two cells of different origin in monoclonal antibody technology. In monoclonal antibody technology, hybridomas are formed by fusing an immortal cell (one that divides continuously) and an antibody-reproducing cell.

HYPOGLYCEMIA. Low blood sugar—the opposite of diabetes.

HYPOTHALAMUS. Brain control area involved in emotions, movement, and eating. Less than the size of a peanut and weighing a quarter of an ounce, this small area deep within the brain also oversees the appetite, blood pressure, sexual behavior, sleep, and emotions and sends orders to the pituitary gland.

HYPOTHALAMUS-PITUITARY-ADRENAL AXIS. The hypothalamus, a section of the brain, sends hormonal messages to the pituitary gland in the center of the skull behind the nose. The pituitary sends hormonal messages to the adrenal glands above the kidneys. Medicines, particularly adrencocorticoids and corticotropin, may affect the communication within this system and cause serious side effects including lowering your resistance to infections.

HYPOTHYROIDISM. Deficiency of thyroid hormone, leading to a slowing down of mental and physical processes.

IL. Interleukins (*see*).

IMMUNE SERUM. Blood serum containing antibodies.

IMMUNE SYSTEM. The cells, biological substances (such as antibodies), and cellular activities that work together to provide resistance to disease.

IMMUNITY. Nonsusceptibility to disease or to the toxic effects of antigenic material.

INFLAMMATORY RESPONSE. Redness, warmth, and swelling produced in response to infection, as the result of increased blood flow and an influx of immune cells and secretions.

INSULIN. A hormone, produced by islet cells of the pancreas gland, essential for metabolism.

INSULIN-LIKE GROWTH FACTOR (IGF). Made mostly in the liver, it has been found to affect bone and connective tissue as well as muscles. It aids nitrogen retention and is being intensively studied in aging research. It interacts with growth hormone (*see*).

INTERFERON (IFN). IFLRA. In 1957, it was discovered that a protein produced naturally by cells could interfere with the ability of a virus to reproduce after it had invaded the body. By the mid-1970s, it appeared that this protein, interferon, might also curtail the spread of certain types of cancer. Genetic engineering enabled the production of sufficient supplies of interferon for experimentation and treatment.

INTERFERON ALFA-2A AND ALFA-2B. Recombinant. Interferons (*see*) are used to treat hairy cell leukemia and AIDS-related Kaposi's sarcoma (*see*). Approved in 1988 for the treatment of genital warts, in 1991 for non-A and non-B hepatitis, and in 1992 for hepatitis B.

INTERFERON GAMMA-1B. An immune-boosting anticancer drug used to treat chronic granulomatous disease, multiple inflammatory tumors. Potential adverse reactions include nausea, vomiting, diarrhea, suppression of bone marrow, headache, chills, fatigue, decreased mental functioning, awkward walking, liver dysfunction, rash, fever, and muscle and joint pain. See INTERFERON.

INTERLEUKINS. In the 1960s, it was discovered that interleukin, a natural substance occurring in the body, transmits signals between types of white blood cells. Interleukin-2 has been used to fight cancers, including melanoma, kidney cancer, and non-Hodgkin's lymphoma, and to stimulate immunity in patients with AIDS. IL-2, originally called T-cell growth factor, is produced in the body T cells (*see*) and has potent effects on the proliferation and differentiation of a number of immune cells. It is on the market to treat a type of kidney cancer. Interleukin-6, which can be protective when produced normally, may destroy bone and cause clotting if overproduced by the body.

IN VITRO. Literally, "in glass." Performed in a laboratory dish or other apparatus.

IN VIVO. In the living organism. Given to humans or animals.

ISCHEMIA. Local deficiency of blood supply, due to spasm or obstruction of an artery.

KAPOSI'S SARCOMA. A rare, malignant skin tumor that occurs in some AIDS patients.

LDL. Low-density lipoprotein cholesterol, the "bad" cholesterol believed to be linked to fat accumulation in the arteries.

LEPTIN. Hormone produced by the obesity gene (ob gene), reported in 1995 to play a part in weight gain.

LEUKOCYTE. White blood cell. A colorless cell in blood, lymph, and tissues that is an important component of the body's immune system.

LH. See LUTEINIZING HORMONE.

LH-RH. Luteinizing hormone–releasing hormone (*see*).

LIBIDO. Psychic energy in general; commonly used to refer to sexual drive.

LIVING SKIN. A bioengineered product using living cells on a matrix to serve as a covering for burns and ulcers and other skin traumas.

LOW BLOOD SUGAR. Hypoglycemia. Less than normal amounts of glucose in circulating blood. Blood sugar naturally drops if we go a long time between meals. Chronic hypoglycemia may be associated with hormonal disorders.

LUPUS. A chronic autoimmune disorder, which means that the immune system attacks the body's own tissues, causing inflammation and damage to multiple organs. There are two types of lupus. Discoid lupus erythematosus especially affects the face, scalp, and neck and causes scarring. Systemic lupus erythematosus is the most serious form and affects many systems of the body.

LUTEINIZING HORMONE (LH). A hormone from the front of the pituitary gland that controls the maturation and function of the ovaries and testes.

LUTEINIZING HORMONE–RELEASING HORMONE (LH-RH). Stimulates secretion of both luteinizing hormone (LH) and follicle-stimulating hormone (FSH). This stimulates the development of eggs in the ovary and their release.

LYMPH. A liquid found within the lymphatic vessels, containing white blood cells and some red blood cells. These cells, collected from tissues throughout the body, flow in the lymphatic vessels through the lymph nodes and eventually into the blood. Lymph is an important part of the body's ability to fight infection and disease.

LYMPH NODES. Small, bean-shaped organs of the immune system, distributed widely throughout the body and linked by lymphatic vessels. Lymph nodes are closets for B, T, and other immune cells.

LYMPHOCYTES. Small white blood cells that are important to the immune system. A decline in lymphocyte function with advancing age is being studied for insights into aging and disease.

LYMPHOKINES. Proteins produced by white blood cells that play a role, as yet not fully understood, in the immune response. See INTERFERON and INTERLEUKINS.

LYMPHOMA. Form of cancer that affects the lymph tissue.

MAO INHIBITORS. See MONOAMINE OXIDASE INHIBITORS.

MEGAKARYOCYTE-STIMULATING FACTOR (MSF). Believed to play a key role in stimulating growth of platelets, elements in the blood that help initiate blood clotting.

MELANIN. A yellow to black pigment that is a factor in skin color.

MELATONIN. This hormone from the pineal gland responds to light and seems to regulate various seasonal changes in the body. As it declines during aging, it may trigger changes throughout the endocrine system.

MENOPAUSE. The time when menstruation stops permanently.

META-ANALYSIS. When researchers evaluate the results of many research studies on a particular subject but do not do the research themselves.

METABOLISM. All biochemical activities carried out by an organism to maintain life.

MONOAMINE OXIDASE INHIBITORS (MAO INHIBITORS). A group of drugs that are used in the treatment of depression and that elevate the level of neurotransmitters by preventing their destruction by enzymes.

MYELIN. White, fatty material that covers most nerves. Degeneration or disappearance of the myelin sheath is characteristic of demyelinating diseases such as multiple sclerosis.

NERVE GROWTH FACTOR (NGF). Believed to maintain and repair nerves.

NEURON. The basic nerve cell of the central nervous system containing a nucleus within the cell body, an axon (a trunklike projection containing neurotransmitters), and dendrites (spiderlike projections that send and receive messages).

NEUROPEPTIDE Y. A neurotransmitter believed to cause carbohydrate craving.

NEUROTRANSMITTERS. Molecules that carry chemical messages between nerve cells. Neurotransmitters are released from nerve cells, diffuse across the minute distance between two nerve cells (synaptic cleft), and bind to a receptor at another nerve site.

NEW DRUG APPLICATION (NDA). Following the completion of all three phases of clinical trials on a new drug intended for public use, the company that produced it files an NDA with the FDA if the data from the trials successfully demonstrates safety and effectiveness. The NDA must contain all the scientific information that has been gathered. NDAs typically run 100,000 pages or more. Originally, by law the FDA was allowed six months to review an NDA. However, in almost all cases, the period between the first submission of an NDA and final FDA approval has exceeded that limit. In 1994, the average NDA review time for new molecular entities approved was nineteen and a half months, down from twenty-six and a half months in 1993 (FDA report, New Drugs Approvals, January 20, 1996). This reduction came at the end of the first year of the agency's new User Fee Program, under which its drug-approval system was redesigned and more reviewers were being trained, financed by fees paid by pharmaceutical companies. See also PHASE I, II, and III, EXPEDITED PROCESS, and FDA APPROVAL.

NGF. Nerve growth factor (*see*).

NIH. National Institutes of Health.

NITRO-. A prefix denoting one atom of nitrogen and two of oxygen.

NITROGEN BALANCE. An expression of the body's protein balance, determined by measurements of nitrogen constituents. If nitrogen intake exceeds excretion, the balance is positive. Excessive retention of nitrogen may indicate kidney disease or other conditions. Negative nitrogen balance may indicate inadequate dietary protein, excessive loss of protein due to goiter, burns, draining wounds, and old age's slowdown of metabolism of protein.

NOREPINEPHRINE. Noradrenaline. A hormone released by the adrenal gland, it has the ability to stimulate that epinephrine does but has minimal inhibitory effects. It has little effect on the lungs, smooth muscles, and metabolic processes and differs from epinephrine in its effect on the heart and blood vessels.

NUCLEIC ACIDS. Large, naturally occurring molecules composed of chemical building blocks known as nucleotides. There are two kinds of nucleic acids, DNA and RNA.

OB GENE. Obesity gene identified by researchers at Rockefeller University in 1994. See LEPTIN.

OPIATES. Narcotics derived from or related to opium such as morphine and codeine.

ORAL CONTRACEPTIVES. Pills that usually consist of synthetic estrogen and progesterone that are taken for three weeks after the last day of a menstrual period. They inhibit ovulation, thereby preventing pregnancy. They have higher levels of the female hormones than found in the hormone replacement compounds for treatment of postmenopausal women.

ORPHAN DRUG. Drugs developed for rare diseases. Congress gave special patent protection to companies developing such medications because of the economics involved.

OSTEOARTHRITIS. A degenerative joint disease of unknown cause. It is characterized by degeneration of the cartilage that lines joints and by the formation of reactive bony outgrowths at the boundary of a joint. This leads to pain and loss of joint function. Osteoarthritis occurs in most people over age sixty.

OSTEOPOROSIS. A condition characterized by low bone mass and an increased susceptibility to bone fractures.

OVULATION. The release of a mature egg cell from the follicle in the ovary in which it develops.

OXYGEN FREE RADICALS. Oxygen molecule with an unpaired electron that is highly reactive, combining readily with other molecules and sometimes causing damage to cells

PANCREAS. A gland composed of two kinds of tissue. One is concerned with internal secretions, or hormones. This tissue is present in the islands or islets of Langerhans where beta cells secrete insulin. Disturbance in insulin production causes metabolic disease, such as diabetes if production is low, and hypoglycemia, low blood sugar, if it puts out too much. The other tissue component of the pancreas produces digestive enzymes.

PARATHYROID (PTH). One of four corners of the thyroid gland (*see*), these pearl-sized glands produce parathyroid hormones, which work with calcitonin from the thyroid gland to control calcium in the blood. A deficiency in this gland causes increased neuromuscular excitability. It is associated with low blood calcium and high blood phosphorus. The disease is due to either accidental removal or damage during removal of the thyroid gland, or to a form of autoimmune disease. Oversecretion of parathyroid hormone results from a tumor, enlargement, or cancer of the glands. This causes high blood levels of calcium, low levels of phosphate and abnormal bone metabolism.

PARKINSON'S DISEASE. Chronic neurologic disease of unknown cause, characterized by tremors, rigidity, and an abnormal gait. The most common variety is Parkinson's disease of unknown cause, or paralysis agitans. Postencephalitic parkinsonism is the diseaselike state occurring after brain inflammation.

PEPTIDE. Two or more amino acids chained together in head-to-tail links. Generally larger than simple amino acids or the monoamines, the largest peptides discovered thus far have forty-four amino acids. Neuropeptides signal the body's endocrine glands to balance salt and water. Opiate peptides can help control pain and anxiety. The peptides work with amino acids. A peptide is present at two ten-thousandths of its partner amino acid or a hundredth the amount of a monoamine.

PERIMENOPAUSE. The time around menopause, usually beginning three to five years before the final period.

PHASE I. These tests take about a year and involve from twenty to eighty normal, healthy volunteers. The tests study a drug's safety profile, including the safe dosage range. The studies also determine how a drug is absorbed, distributed, metabolized, and excreted, and the duration of its action.

PHASE II. In this phase, controlled studies of approximately 100 to 300 volunteer patients (people with the disease the drug being tested is created to treat) assess the drug's effectiveness, which takes about two years.

PHASE III. This phase lasts about three years and usually involves 1,000 to 3,000 patients in clinics and hospitals. Physicians monitor patients closely to determine efficacy of the drug and identify adverse reactions to it. Private "study centers" are replacing university research facilities for testing new pharmaceuticals, a new development in drug testing. The private centers, which advertise for patients over the radio, offer a more rapid, less expensive means of clinical trials. Questions about the selection of substances to be tested and the quality of research by non-university investigators remain to be answered. See also NEW DRUG APPLICATION and EXPEDITED PROCESS.

PINEAL GLAND. A cone-shaped structure about the size of a pea that lies very nearly in the center of the brain. Once thought to be a left-over from some earlier age of mankind, it is now believed to be a biological clock. It produces melatonin (*see*).

PITUITARY GLAND. The pea-sized gland situated at the base of the brain, once thought to be the master gland that gave "orders" to other glands. It is now known that the pituitary gland takes its orders from the hypothalamus (*see*). The pituitary then sends out orders to the other glands in the body. The frontal lobe of the gland produces growth hormone, which regulates growth; prolactin, which stimulates the breasts and has other functions as yet not clearly understood; and hormones that stimulate the thyroid, adrenals, ovaries, and testes. The back lobe of the pituitary produces antidiuretic hormone, which acts on the kidneys and regulates urine output, and oxytocin, which stimulates the contractions of the womb during childbirth.

PLACEBO. A chemically inactive substance used as a comparison during studies to determine how effective an active substance is. A placebo may also be given to a patient to relieve a condition that does not require a medication. The "placebo effect" may occur when the patient, believing he or she has received a real medication, releases self-made tranquilizers or stimulants and actually changes internal secretions as if an active pharmaceutical had been given.

PLANT ESTROGENS. A host of estrogens have been identified in plants. Although they are considerably less active than those in animals, chronic exposure may lead to the accumulation of levels that are active in humans.

PLAQUE. Tiny patches or unnatural formations on tissues. Atheroma plaques, which are found in walls of arteries, contain some fats and scar tissue.

PLASMA. The fluid portion of the blood or lymph that carries in solution a wide range of ions, minerals, vitamins, antibodies, proteins, enzymes, and/or other essential substances.

PLATELETS. Colorless, small disks found in blood that aid in clotting.

PRECURSOR. A substance that turns into another active or more mature substance. Beta-carotene is a precursor of vitamin A because the body can use it to make vitamin A.

PREMENSTRUAL TENSION. Cyclic occurrence of emotional symptoms associated with body changes about a week before onset of the menstrual period. Includes physical symptoms such as abdominal bloating, weight gain, puffiness, and tenderness of the breasts.

PRIAPISM. Persistent erection of the penis, accompanied by pain and tenderness.

PROGESTERONE. One of the female sex hormones produced by the ovaries.

PROGESTIN. The synthetic form of progesterone.

PROLACTIN. A hormone secreted by the front lobe of the pituitary gland that stimulates production of milk and may have other activities not yet identified.

PROSTAGLANDINS. A group of extremely potent hormonelike substances that occur in minute amounts in virtually all body tissues.

PROTEINS. Molecules made up of amino acids arranged in a specific order determined by the genetic code. Proteins are essential for all life processes. Certain ones such as the enzymes that protect against free radicals and the lymphokines produced in the immune system are being studied extensively by gerontologists.

PSORIASIS. A chronic disease of the skin of unknown cause, characterized by elevated, silvery lesions, often on the elbows, knees, scalp, and lower back. Related to arthritis.

RECEPTOR. A protein molecule that may also be composed of fat and carbohydrate that resides on the surface or in the nucleus of a cell and recognizes and binds a specific molecule of appropriate size, shape, and charge. Receptors are activated by specific nerve chemicals, hormones, or drugs and can be regarded as "biological locks" that can be "opened" only with specific keys.

RECEPTOR BINDING ASSAY. A technique to determine the presence and amount of a drug, neurotransmitter, or receptor in a biological system.

RECOMBINANT DNA. The DNA formed by combining segments of DNA from different types of organisms. Recombinant DNA technology is one technique of genetic engineering.

RELEASING FACTORS. Produced by the hypothalamus and then sent to the pituitary, where they cause the release of appropriate hormones. Among those that have been found are luteinizing hormone–releasing hormone (LH-RH), which affects the release of the sex hormones, and thyroid hormone–releasing factor (TH-RF), which affects the release of the thyroid hormone. Both LH-RH and TH-RF have behavioral effects. LH-RH, for example, enhances mating behavior. TH-RF can cause stimulation.

RHEUMATOID ARTHRITIS. A type of arthritis that particularly attacks the small joints of the hands, wrists, and feet. The joints become painful, swollen, stiff, and in severe cases, deformed. This autoimmune disorder usually starts in early adulthood or middle age and affects two to three times more women than men.

RIBONUCLEIC ACID (RNA). A molecule similar to DNA that functions primarily to decode the instructions for protein manufacture that are carried by genes.

RNA. Ribonucleic acid (*see*).

SEBACEOUS GLAND. Secretes oil.

SEROLOGY. Study of blood serum and reactions between the antibodies and antigens in the blood.

SEROTONIN. A natural neurotransmitter (chemical messenger between nerve cells) in the brain. Low levels are associated with depression, and some antidepressants seem to work by triggering increased production of serotonin. The substance also plays a role in temperature regulation and sleep. It is believed that it can be raised by eating carbohydrates. Inhibits secretions in the digestive tract and stimulates smooth muscles. It is an important regulator of mood and affects appetite. It may be useful for victims of seasonal depression, people who want to stop smoking, and others.

SERUM. The clear portion of the blood, separated from its solid elements.

SET POINT. Adipostat. Located in the brain, it is a biological mechanism that powerfully resists changes in body fat and body weight attempted by diet and exercise. It returns the body to the original weight.

SHINGLES. See HERPES VARICELLA ZOSTER.

SOMATOPAUSE. The name given the decline in aging of growth hormone, which results in diminished lean-body mass, increased fat deposits, and osteoporosis. Kidney function declines, and sleep disturbances are common.

SOMATOTROPIN. See HUMAN GROWTH HORMONE.

STEM CELLS. Cells from which all blood cells derive.

STEROIDS. Class of compounds including some of hormonal origin, such as cortisone, used to treat the inflammations caused by allergies. Cholesterol, precursors of certain vitamins, bile acids, alcohols, and many plant derivatives such as digitalis are steroids. Steroids can reduce white blood cell production and reduce prostaglandins and leukotrienes. Natural and synthetic steroids have four rings of carbon atoms but have different actions according to what is attached to the rings. Cortisone and oral contraceptives are steroids.

STRESS. Mental or physical tension within resulting from a person's response to physical, chemical, or emotional factors. Stress can refer to physical exertion as well as mental anxiety.

SUPPRESSOR T CELLS. A subset of T cells that can turn off antibody production and other immune responses.

SYMPATHETIC NERVOUS SYSTEM. One of the major divisions of the autonomic nervous system; it regulates involuntary muscle actions such as the beating of the heart and breathing. The sympathetic nerves that leave the brain and spinal cord pass through the nerve cell clusters (ganglia) and are distributed to the heart, lungs, intestines, blood vessels, and sweat glands. In general, sympathetic nerves dilate the pupils, constrict small blood vessels, and increase heart rate. They are the nerves that prepare us for fight or flight. Parasympathetic nerves, the other part of the autonomic system, slow things down after you stop exercising or the danger has passed. The system also involves circulating substances produced by the adrenal glands.

SYNAPSE. The minute space between two neurons or between a neuron and an organ across which nerve impulses are chemically transmitted.

SYNDROME. A set of symptoms that occur together and collectively characterize a disease or condition.

T CELLS. White blood cells that are developed in the thymus gland (*see*) and play a vital part in immunity.

TESTOSTERONE. The male hormone, it is produced in the testes and may decline with age, though less than estrogen in women. Researchers are investigating its ability to strengthen muscles and prevent frailty and disability in older men when administered as testosterone therapy.

THYMIC HUMORAL FACTOR (THF). A natural hormone isolated from calf thymus, it reportedly increases the number of T lymphocytes and increases immunity in those with weakened or absent defenses.

THYMOPENTIN. Timunox. A biologically active substance similar to the thymus (*see*) hormone thymopoietin. It is being developed for the treatment of HIV infections in people who have not yet shown the symptoms of AIDS.

THYMOSIN A-1. A substance from the thymus gland (*see*) that is being tested against chronic active hepatitis B and C, viral infections that affect the liver.

THYMOSTIMULIN (TP2). A substance from the thymus that has shown to have some slight promise against head and neck squamous-cell carcinoma by Dutch researchers, but the work is too early yet to supply definitive answers.

THYMUS GLAND. An organ in the chest that helps to activate the body's defenses against infection.

THYROID. The thyroid is a butterfly-shaped gland located in the neck with a "wing" on either side of the windpipe. The gland produces thyroxine, which controls the rates of chemical reactions in the body. Generally, the more thyroxine, the faster the body works. Thyroxine needs iodine to function.

THYROID-STIMULATING HORMONE (TSH). A hormone from the front part of the pituitary gland that stimulates the thyroid gland (*see*).

THYROTROPIN-RELEASING HORMONE (TRH). Stimulates the pituitary to release a hormone that chemically stimulates the thyroid gland into releasing its hormone. TRH was reported in 1996 to have shown effectiveness in helping to combat nerve damage in animals, and in a small clinical study of patients with spinal cord injury, it was reported as promising.

TISSUE ENGINEERING. The engineering of individual cells to form structures that carry out the functions of normal tissue. Grafts of "living skin" made in the laboratory are an example.

T LYMPHOCYTES. See T CELLS.

TRANQUILIZER. A popular term used to describe drugs such as Valium that depress the central nervous system to produce calming and sedative effects.

TRANSFORMING GROWTH FACTOR (TGFs). These play a part in wound repair and help bones grow. They are active in blood-vessel formation and are believed to inhibit tumors.

TRANSGENIC ORGANISM. An organism formed by the insertion of foreign genetic material into the germ line cells of organisms. Recombinant DNA techniques are commonly used to produce transgenic organisms.

TRYPTOPHAN. Trofan. Trypatcin. A tremendous amount of research is now in progress with this amino acid (*see*). First isolated in milk in 1901, it is now being studied as a means to calm hyperactive children, induce sleep, and fight depression and pain. Although it is sold over the counter, tryptophan is not believed to be completely harmless and has been suspected of being a cocarcinogen (abets a cancer-causing agent) and of affecting the liver when taken in high doses. As with niacin, it is capable of preventing and curing pellagra. It is used by the body to make the brain hormone serotonin and is indispensable for the manufacture of certain cell proteins.

TSH. Thyroid-stimulating hormone (*see*).

VACCINE. A substance that contains the antigen of an organism and that stimulates active immunity and future protection against infection by the organism.

WHITE BLOOD CELLS. See LEUKOCYTES.

INTRODUCTION

1. Richard Hodes, Vicky Cahan, and Marcia Pruzan, "The National Institute on Aging at Its Twentieth Anniversary: Achievements and Promise of Research on Aging," *American Geriatrics Society Journal* 44, no. 2 (February 1996): 204–6.

2. *Bureau of Census Report 65+ in the United States* (Washington, D.C., May 20, 1996).

3. Phyllis Moen, "Limbo—a New Life Stage for Americans Who Retire Earlier but Live Longer" (paper presented at the American Association for the Advancement of Science, Baltimore, Md., February 12, 1996).

1: THE CHEMICALS THAT CONTROL YOUR RIPENING

1. "Pharmacologic Treatment of Acute Traumatic Brain Injury," *Journal of the American Medical Association* 276, no. 7 (August 21, 1996): 569–70.

2: STRESS AND MAINTAINING YOUTHFUL IMMUNITY

1. J. D. Ratcliff, "How to Avoid Harmful Stress," *Today's Health,* July 1970, 42–44.

2. "How We Respond to Fear and Stress," in *Reader's Digest ABC's of the Human Mind,* ed. Alma E. Guinness (Pleasantville, N.Y.: Reader's Digest Association Books, 1987), 84–85.

3. Albert Maisel, *The Hormone Quest* (New York: Random House, 1965).

4. "Adreno-corticosteroids," *Arthritis Foundation Report* (May 1974).

5. "Dehydroepiandrosterone—Therapeutic Use," *Time,* 1995, electronic collection: A16043871.

6. N. Orentreich et al.,"Age Changes and Sex Differences in Serum Dehydroepiandrosterone Sulfate Concentrations Throughout

Adulthood," *Journal of Clinical Endocrinology and Metabolism* 59 (1984): 551.

7. E. Barrett-Connor et al., "A Prospective Study of Dehydroepi-androsterone Sulfate Mortality and Cardiovascular Disease," *New England Journal of Medicine* 315 (1986): 1519–24.

8. H. Iano et al., "Chemoprevention by dietary dehydroepiandros-terone against promotion/progression phase of radiation-induced mammary tumorigenesis in rats," *Journal of Steroid Biochemistry and Molecular Biology* 54, no. 1–2 (July 1995): 47–53.

9. William Regelson, Mohammed Kalimi, and Roger Loria, "De-hydroepiandrosterone (DHEA): The Precursor Steroid: Introductory Remarks," in *The Biologic Role of Dehydroepiandrosterone (DHEA)*, eds. M. Kalimi and W. Regelson (New York: Walter de Gruyter, 1990), 1–6.

10. Ann Guidici Fettner, "DHEA gets respect," *Harvard Health Letter* 19, no. 9 (1994): 1.

11. A. D. Schwartz, D. K. Fairman, and L. L. Pashko, "The Bio-logical Significance of Dehydroepiandrosterone," in *Biologic Role of Dehydroepiandrosterone*, 7–11.

12. Barrett-Connor et al., "Prospective Study of Dehydro-epiandrosterone."

13. E. E. Balieu, "Studies on Dehydroepiandrosterone (DHEA) and Its Sulphate During Aging," *Comptes Rendus de l'Académie des Sciences*, 3d ser., *Sciences de la Vie* 328, no. 1 (January 1995): 7–11.

14. A. J. Morales et al., "Effects of replacement dose of dehydro-epiandrosterone in men and women of advancing age," *Journal of Clinical Endocrinology and Metabolism* 78, no. 6 (June 1994).

15. S. S. Yen, A. J. Morales, and O. Khorram, "Replacement of DHEA in aging men and women. Potential remedial effects," *Annals of the New York Academy of Sciences* 774 (December 29, 1995): 128–42.

16. Burkhard Bilger, "Forever Young," *Sciences*, September/ October 1995, 26–29.

17. William Regelson, Roger Loria, and Mohammed Kalimi, "Dehydroepiandrosterone (DHEA)—the 'Mother Steroid,'" *Annals of the New York Academy of Sciences* 719 (1994): 543–51.

18. William Regelson and Mohammed Kalimi, "Dehydroepiandrosterone (DHEA)—the Multifunctional Steroid," *Annals of the New York Academy of Sciences* 719 (1994).

19. William Regelson, and M. Kalimi, "Preface," in *Biologic Role of Dehydroepiandrosterone*.

20. Raymond Daynes, personal communication with author, August 21, 1996.

21. Thomas Evans, personal communication with author, August 22, 1996.

22. G. M. Rubanyi, "Vascular Effects of Oxygen-Derived Free Radicals," *Free Radical Biological Medicine* 4 (1988): 107–20.

23. C. R. Merill, M. G. Harrington, and T. Sunderland, "Reduced Plasma Dehydroepiandrosterone Concentration in HIV Infections and Alzheimer's Disease," in *Biologic Role of Dehydroepiandrosterone,* 102–3.

24. J. Y. Yang, A. Schwartz, and E. E. Henderson, "Inhibition of 3'azido-3'deoxythymidine–resistant HIV-1 infection by dehydroepiandrosterone in vitro," *Biochemistry and Biophysics Research* 201, no. 3 (June 30, 1994): 1424–32.

25. T. S. Dyner et al., "An open-label dose-escalation trial of oral dehydroepiandrosterone tolerance and pharmacokinetics in patients with HIV disease," *Journal of Acquired Immune Deficiency Syndrome* 6, no. 5 (May 1993): 459–65.

26. R. F. van Vollenhoven, E. G. Engleman, and J. L. McGuire, "An open study of dehydroepiandrosterone in systemic lupus erythematosus," *Arthritic and Rheumatism* 37, no. 9 (September 1994): 1305–10.

27. T. Suzuki et al., "Low serum levels of dehydroepiandrosterone may cause deficient IL-2 production by lymphocytes in patients with systemic lupus erythematosus," *Clinical Experimental Immunology* 99, no. 2 (February 1995): 251–55.

28. A. Winter and R. Winter, "Arthritis," in *Free Medical Information by Phone and by Mail* (Prentice Hall, 1993), 27.

29. G. M. Hall, L. A. Perry, and T. D. Spector, "Depressed levels of dehydroepiandrosterone sulphate in postmenopausal women with rheumatoid arthritis but no relation with axial bone density," *Annals of Rheumatic Disease* 52, no. 3 (March 1993): 211–14.

30. S. Miklos et al., "Dehydroepiandrosterone sulphate in the diagnosis of osteoporosis," *Acta Biomedical Ateno Parmense* 66, no. 3–4 (1995): 139–46.

31. E. Barrett-Connor, D. Kritz-Silverstein, and S. L. Edelstein, "A prospective study of dehydroepiandrosterone sulfate (DHEA-S) and bone mineral density in older men and women," *American Journal of Epidemiology* 137, no. 2 (January 15, 1993): 201–6.

32. J. R. Williams of Temple University, "(DHEA) Derivatives That Protect Against Cancer, Obesity, Diabetes, and Slow Down Aging" (paper presented at American Chemical Society meeting, Miami Beach, Fl., September 10, 1989); H. Inano et al., "Chemoprevention by dietary dehydroepiandrosterone"; "Antiaging Drug Linked to Cancer," *Cancer Biotechnology Weekly,* January 15, 1996, 1.

33. William Regelson, Mohammed Kalimi, and Roger Loria, "DHEA: Some Thoughts as to Its Biologic and Clinical Action," in *Biologic Role of Dehydroepiandrosterone,* 405–45.

34. Ibid.

35. J. Sonka and M. Stravkova, "Survival of irradiated mice pretreated by dehydroepiandrosterone," *Agressologie* 5 (1970): 421–26.

36. Regelson, Kalimi, and Loria, "DHEA: Some Thoughts," 405–45.

37. Ibid.

38. Arthur Schwartz, *American Journal of Medicine* 98, no. 1A (January 16, 1995): 405–475.

39. Regelson and Kalimi, "Dehydroepiandrosterone (DHEA)—the Multifunctional Steroid," 564–71.

40. Richard Podell, personal communication with author, August 12, 1996.

41. Arthur Schwartz, personal communication with author, August 21, 1996.

42. Ibid.

43. Bruce Hirsch and Marc Weksler, "Normal Changes in Host Defense," in *Merck Manual of Geriatrics* (Rahway, N.J., 1990), 877–78.

44. Ibid.

45. Joseph Prous, *The Year's Drug News: Therapeutic Targets* (Barcelona, Spain: Prous Science Publishers, 1994), 360.

46. Ibid.

47. Naomi Judd, *Love Can Build a Bridge* (New York: Villard Books, 1993).

48. J. D. Kerrebijn et al., "In vivo effects of thymostimulin treatment on monocyte polarization, dendritic cell clustering and serum p15E-like transmembrane factors in operable head and neck squamous cell carcinoma patients," *European Archives of Otorhinolaryngology* 252, no. 7 (1995): 409–16.

49. B. A. Farhat et al., "Evaluation of the efficacy and safety of thymus humoral factor–gamma 2 in the management of chronic hepatitis B," *Journal of Hepatology* 23, no. 1 (July 1995): 21–27.

50. A. R. Saha, E. M. Hadden, and J. W. Hadden, "Zinc induces thymulin secretion from human thymic epithelial cells in vitro and augments splenocyte and thymocyte responses in vivo," *International Journal of Immunopharmacology* 17, no. 9 (September 1995): 729–33.

51. William Weigle, "Effects of Aging on the Immune System," *Hospital Practice,* December 15, 1989, 112–16.

3: GROWTH HORMONES

1. Maisel, *Hormone Quest,* 238.

2. Ibid.

3. William Abrams, Robert Berkow, and Andrew Fletcher, eds., *Merck Manual of Geriatrics* (Rahway, N.J.: Merck & Co., 1990), 946.

4. Harold Schmeck Jr., "Human Growth Hormone Made by Bacteria: Tests in Patients Next Step in Several Diseases," *New York Times,* January 6, 1981, C1.

5. Eli Lilly and Company announcement, Indianapolis, Ind., August 7, 1996.

6. Andrew Hoffman, Steven Lieberman, and Gian Paolo Ceda, "Growth Hormone Therapy in the Elderly: Implications for the Aging," *Psychoneuroendocrinology* 17, no. 4 (1992): 327–33.

7. Jake Powrie, Andrew Weissberger, and P. Sonksen, "Growth Hormone Replacement Therapy for Growth Hormone–Deficient Adults," Review Articles, *Drugs* 49, no. 5 (1995): 656–63.

8. L. Sacca, A. Cittadini, and S. Fazio, "Growth Hormone and the Heart," *Endocrinology Review* 15 (1994): 555–73; L. Sacca and S. Fazio, "Cardiac Performance: growth hormone enters the race," *National Medical Journal* 2 (1996): 29–31.

9. S. Fazio et al., "A Preliminary Study of Growth Hormone in the Treatment of Dilated Cardiomyopathy," *New England Journal of Medicine* 334 (1996): 809–14.

10. Correspondence to *New England Journal of Medicine* 335, no. 9 (August 29, 1996): 672–74.

11. University of Washington release, March 23, 1993.

12. R. S. Schwartz, "Trophic Factor Supplementation: effect on the age-associated changes in body composition," *Journal of Gerontology and Biological Science* 50 (November 1995): 151–56.

13. Robert Schwartz, personal communication with author, August 27, 1996.

14. M. A. Bach, M. Thorner, et al., "An Orally Active Growth Hormone Secretagogue (MK-677) Increases Pulsatile GH Secretion and Circulating IGF-1 in the Healthy Elderly" (paper presented at 10th International Congress of Endocrinology, San Francisco, Calif., June 12–15, 1996).

15. Merck Annual Report 1995 and other material from Merck, August 27, 1996.

16. Marc Blackman, personal communication with author, August 24, 1996.

17. Jens Jorgensen et al., "Three years of growth hormone treatment in growth hormone–deficient adults: near normalization of body composition and physical performance," *European Journal of Endocrinology* 130 (1994): 224–28.

18. Ibid.

19. K. Brixen et al., "Short term treatment with growth hormone stimulates osteoblastic and osteoclastic activity in osteopenic postmenopausal women: a dose response study," *Journal of Bone Mineral Research* 10, no. 12 (December 1995): 1865–74.

20. Kevin E. Yarasheski et al., "Effect of Growth Hormone and Resistance Exercise on Muscle Growth and Strength in Older Men," *American Journal of Physiology,* March 1994, 268.

21. Maxine Papadakis et al., "Growth Hormone Replacement in Healthy Older Men Improves Body Composition but Not Functional Ability," *Annals of Internal Medicine* 124 (April 15, 1996): 708–16.

22. Marc Blackman, personal communication with author, August 20, 1996.

23. L. Cohen et al., "Carpal tunnel syndrome and gynaecomastia during growth hormone treatment of elderly men with low circulation IFG-I concentrations," *Clinical Endocrinology* 39 (1993): 417–25.

24. Beth Howard, "Growing Younger: Can Growth Hormone Make the Clock Run Backwards?" *Longevity,* October 1992, 40.

25. Laura Johannes, "Serano Wins Approval for AIDS Drug," *Wall Street Journal,* August 27, 1996, B4.

26. Dana Reisman, personal communication with author, June 21, 1996.

27. Michael Thorner, personal communication with author, August 28, 1996.

4: GROWTH FACTORS

1. E. Pennisi, "Gene gun, growth factors promote healing," *Science News* 146, no. 14 (October 1, 1994): 213.

2. Sabine Werner et al., "The Function of KGF in Morphogenesis

of Epithelium and Reepithelialization of Wounds," *Science* 266, no. 5186 (November 4, 1994): 819.

3. Rachel Nowak, "Moving developmental research into the clinic (Frontiers in Biology: Development)," *Science* 266, no. 5185 (October 28, 1994): 567.

4. Michael McCarthy, "Bioengineered tissue moves toward the clinic," *Lancet* 348 (August 17, 1996): 466.

5. "Spotlight on Research: Tissue Engineering Research Aims to Create Artificial Organs," *Industry Collegium Report* (MIT) (May 1996): 5.

6. Lia Unrau, "Tissue Engineered Skin to Be First of Many Products," Rice University news release, August 6, 1996.

7. E. Corpas, S. M. Harman, and M. R. Blackman, "Human Growth Hormone and Human Aging," *Endocrinology Review* 14, no. 1 (February 1993): 20–39.

8. Hoffman, Lieberman, and Paolo Ceda, "Growth Hormone Therapy in the Elderly."

9. V. Hesse et al., "Insulin-like growth factor I correlations to changes of the hormonal status in puberty and age," *Experimental Clinical Endocrinology* 102, no. 4 (1994): 289–98.

10. A. V. Nall et al., "Transforming growth factor beta-1 improves wound healing and random flap survival in normal and irradiated rats," *Archives of Otolaryngology Head and Neck Surgery* (February 1996), 171–77; T. I. Morales, "Transforming growth factor-beta and insulin-like growth factor-1 restore proteoglycan metabolism of bovine articular cartilage," *Archives of Biochemistry and Biophysics* 315 (November 15, 1994): 190–98.

11. C. Missale et al., "Nerve growth factor in the anterior pituitary localization in mammotroph cells and cosecretion with prolactin by dopamine regulated mechanism," *Proceedings of the National Academy of Sciences, USA* 93, no. 9 (April 30, 1996): 4240–45.

12. K. S. Chen et al., "Synaptic loss in cognitively impaired aged rats is ameliorated by chronic human nerve growth factor infusion," *Neuroscience* 68, no. 1 (September 1995): 19–27; J. D. Cooper et al.,

"Reduced transport of nerve growth factor by cholinergic neurons and down-regulated TrkA expression in the medial septum of aged rats," *Neuroscience* 62, no. 3 (October 1994): 625–29; K. Ohnishi et al., "Age-related decrease of nerve growth factor–like immunoreactivity in the basal forebrain of senescence-accelerated mice," *Acta Neuropathology* 90, no. 1 (1995): 11–16.

13. A. L. Markowska, D. Price, and V. S. Koliatrsos, "Selective effects of nerve growth factor on spatial recent memory as assessed by a delayed nonmatching-to-position task in the water maze," *Journal of Neuroscience* 16, no. 10 (May 15, 1996): 3541–48.

14. Carolyn McNeil, "Alzheimer's Disease: Unraveling the Mystery," National Institute on Aging, NIH Publication No. 95-3782, October 1995, 32.

15. Hodes, Cahan, and Pruzan, "The National Institute on Aging at Its Twentieth Anniversary," 204–6.

16. Rebecca Hughes, "Brain Repair: Rewiring the Mind," *Longevity,* December 1992, 14.

17. J. M. Simard et al., "Ionic channel currents in cultured neurons from human cortex," *Journal of Neuroscience Research* 34, no. 2 (February 1, 1993): 170–78; K. N. Westlund et al., "NGF producing transfected 3T3 cells: behavioral and histological assessment of transplants in nigra lesioned rats," *Journal of Neurosciences* 41, no. 3 (June 15, 1995): 367–73; Hughes, "Brain Repair," 14.

18. Christopher Reeve, *Today Show,* August 26, 1996.

19. W. A. Bauman et al., "Blunted growth hormone response to intravenous arginine in subjects with spinal cord injury," *Hormone Metabolism Research* 26, no. 3 (March 1994), 152–56.

20. K. R. Shetty et al., "Studies of growth hormone/insulin-like growth factor-1 in polio survivors," *Annals of the New York Academy of Science* 753 (May 25, 1995): 276–84.

21. C. C. Stichel et al., "Clearance of myelin constitutents and axonal sprouting on the transected postcommissural fornix of the adult rat," *European Journal of Neuroscience* 7, no. 3 (March 1, 1995): 401–11.

22. T. Sivron, M. E. Schwab, and M. Schwartz, "Presence of growth inhibitors in fish optic nerve myelin: post injury changes," *Journal of Neurology* 343, no. 2 (May 8, 1994): 237–46.

23. D. T. Villareal and J. E. Morley, "Trophic Factors in Aging. Should Older People Receive Hormonal Replacement Therapy?" *Drugs and Aging* 4, no. 6 (June 1994): 492–509.

24. Richard Davey, "Interleukin-2 Injections Produce Dramatic, Sustained Increase in CD4+ T Cells in Patients with Early HIV Infection" (paper presented at the International Conference on AIDS, Vancouver, British Columbia, July 10, 1996).

25. John Hamilton, "Rheumatoid arthritis: opposing actions of haemopoietic growth factors and slow-acting anti-rheumatic drugs," *Lancet* 342, no. 8870 (August 28, 1993): 536.

26. Y. Masuda et al., "Platelet-derived growth factor B-chain homodimer suppressing a convulsion of epilepsy model mouse E1," *Biochemistry and Biophysics Research* 223, no. 1 (June 5, 1996): 60–63.

27. Meyer Davidson, "Carbohydrate Metabolism and Diabetes Mellitus," in *Merck Manual of Geriatrics,* 790–91.

28. Gregg Adams and Donald Dafoe, "Potential New Diabetes Treatment Using Pancreas Cells and Growth Factor IGF-1" (paper presented at the American Society of Transplant Surgeons Annual Meeting, Dallas, Tex., May 30, 1996).

29. M. A. Bach, S. Chin, and C. A. Bondy, "The effects of subcutaneous insulin-like growth factor-I infusion in insulin-dependent diabetes mellitus," *Journal of Clinical Endocrinology and Metabolism* 79, no. 4 (October 1994): 1040–45.

30. Gina Kolata, "Gene Therapy Shows First Signs of Bypassing Arterial Blockage," *New York Times,* August 27, 1996, C3; Jeffrey Isner and L. J. Feldman, "Gene Therapy for Arterial Disease," *Lancet* 344, no. 8938 (December 17, 1994): 1653–54; Jeffrey Isner, "Clinical evidence of angiogenesis after arterial gene transfer of phVEG F165 in patients with ischemic limb," *Lancet* 348, no. 9024 (August 10, 1996): 370–74.

31. Dorothy Bonn, "Blocking angiogenesis in diabetic retinopathy," *Lancet,* August 31, 1996, 604.

32. H. G. Garg et al., "Antiproliferative role of 3-0-sulfate glucosamine in heparin on cultured pulmonary artery smooth muscle cells," *Biochemical and Biophysical Research* 224, no. 2 (July 16, 1996): 468–73; A. Skaletz-Rorowski et al., "Heparin induced overexpression of basic fibroblast growth factor," *Arteriosclerosis and Thrombosis Vascular Biology* 16, no. 8 (August 1996): 1063–69; M. A. Palmeri et al., "The role of heparin sulfate in the treatment of pregnant women with circulatory deficiency syndrome," *Minerva Gynecology* 48 no. 3 (March 1996): 119–23; H. Akimoto et al., "Heparin and heparin sulfate block angiotensin II–induced hypertrophy in cultured neonatal rat cardiomyocytes," *Circulation* 93 no. 4 (February 15, 1996): 810–16.

33. Patricia Forsyth, "UC–San Francisco Researchers Find New Clue to Liver Regeneration," University of San Francisco news report, July 9, 1987, based on May 1987 issue of *Gastroenterology.*

34. A. Kahn et al., "Age-related bone loss. A hypothesis and initial assessment in mice," *Clinical Orthopedics* 313 (April 1995): 69–75; Villareal and Morley, "Trophic Factors in Aging."

35. Mark Quinn, "Hormone Hope for Gut Disease Treatment," *Lancet* 348 (August 3, 1996): 325.

36. Hamilton, "Rheumatoid arthritis," 536.

37. Barry Eppley, personal communication with author, August 8, 1996.

5: THIN WITHIN—HORMONAL CONTROL OF WEIGHT AS THE YEARS GO BY

1. JoAnn Manson et al., "Body Weight and Longevity: A Reassessment," *Journal of the American Medical Association* 257 no. 3 (January 16, 1987): 353–58.

2. S. Roberts and P. Fuss, "Older men don't burn as many calories after overeating as their younger counterparts," Quarterly Report, U.S. Department of Agriculture, January-March 1996, 11.

3. Ronald D. Cape, "Malnutrition, Weight Loss, and Anorexia," in *Merck Manual of Geriatrics,* 4–12.

4. "Eating Right to Make the Most of Maturity," Ross Laboratories, June 1991.

5. Denise Mann, "Menopausal Women at Risk of Weight Gain," *Medical Tribune News Service,* November 9, 1995.

6. Donna Kritz-Silverstein and Elizabeth Barrett-Connor, "Long-term Estrogen Use Does Not Cause Weight Gain," *Journal of the American Medical Association* (January 2, 1996).

7. M. W. Schwartz et al., "Cerebrospinal Fluid Leptin Levels: Relationship to Plasma Levels and to Adiposity in Humans," *National Medicine* 5 (May 2, 1996): 589–93.

8. Abrams, Berkow, and Fletcher, *Merck Manual of Geriatrics,* 783.

9. P. A. Singer, Paul W. Ladenson, et al., "Treatment Guidelines for Patients with Hypothyroidism," *Journal of the American Medical Association* (July 24, 1996).

10. "Graves' Disease—A Varied Picture," *Lahey Clinic Health Letter,* July 1991, 1–2.

11. Abrams, Berkow, and Fletcher, *Merck Manual of Geriatrics,* 77.

12. Lawrence Altman, "A White House Puzzle: Immunity Ailments," *New York Times,* May 28, 1991, 1.

13. Ibid.

14. A. Ensminger et al., eds., *Concise Encyclopedia of Foods and Nutrition* (Boca Raton, Florida: CRC Press, 1995), 783.

15. National Institutes of Health, "Diet and Exercise in Noninsulin-Dependent Diabetes Mellitus," Consensus Development Conference Statement, Vol. 6, no. 8 (December 10, 1986).

16. E. Coleman et al., "Weight Loss Reduces Abdominal Fat and Improves Insulin Action in Middle-aged and Older Men with Impaired Glucose Tolerance," *Metabolism* no. 11 (November 1995): 1502–8.

17. Abrams, Berkow, and Fletcher, *Merck Manual of Geriatrics,* 1186.

18. Ibid., 793–94.

19. "Insulin May Not Be the Only Answer to Diabetes" (American Chemical Society release, Washington, D.C., June 10, 1996).

20. Ibid.

21. M. A. Pereira et al., "Physical Inactivity and Glucose Tolerance in the Multiethnic Island of Mauritius," *Medical Science Sport Exercise* 27, no. 12 (December 1995): 1626–34.

22. D. J. Evans et al., "Relationship of Androgenic Activity to Adipocyte Morphology and Insulin Resistance in Premenopausal Women" (paper presented at the 65th Annual Meeting of the Endocrine Society, San Antonio, Tex., June 10, 1983).

23. Manson, "Body Weight and Longevity."

24. Arthur Winter and Ruth Winter, *Eat Right Be Bright* (New York: St. Martin's Press, 1988), 230.

25. Renee Twombly, "Morbid Obesity Has Roots in Hormonal Imbalance, Duke Physician Tells NIH," *Duke University News,* August 1, 1991.

26. Theresa Tamkins, "Brain Hormone Found to Stimulate Appetite," *Medical Tribune News Service,* March 20, 1996.

6: MELATONIN

1. J. de Mairan, *"Observation botanique,"* in *Histoire de l'Académie Royale des Sciences,* 35–36.

2. E. D. Weitzman, "Circadian rhythms and episodic hormone secretion in man," *Annual Review of Medicine* 27 (1976): 225–43; E. D. Weitzman et al., "Twenty-four-hour pattern of the episodic secretion of cortisol in normal subjects," *Journal of Clinical Endocrinology and Metabolism* 33 (1971): 14–22.

3. Martin C. Moore-Ede, Frank Sulzman, and Charles Fuller, *The Clocks That Time Us, Physiology of the Circadian Timing Systems* (Cambridge, Mass.: Harvard University Press, 1982).

4. S. W. Stanbury and A. E. Thomson, "Diurnal variations in electrolyte excretion," *Clinical Science and Molecular Medicine* 10 (1951): 267–93.

5. Theresa Tamkins, "When Treating Some Diseases, Timing Is Everything," *Medical Tribune News Service,* February 29, 1996.

6. Lydia Dotto, "At the Very Root of Our Existence Lies the Complex Tapestry of Circadian Rhythmicity," *Journal of Addiction Research Foundation,* February 1, 1990, 12.

7. Judith Willis, "Keeping Time to Circadian Rhythms," *FDA Consumer,* July/August 1990, 19–21.

8. S. M. Reppert et al., "Putative melatonin receptors in a human biological clock," *Science* 242 (1988): 78.

9. George Bray, "Melatonin—the Hormone of Darkness," *New England Journal of Medicine* 327, no. 19 (November 5, 1992): 1377–78.

10. "Night Workers' Body Clocks Always out of Sync, Studies Show," *Journal of the American Sleep Disorders Association and the Sleep Research Society,* October 1992.

11. Bray, "Melatonin," 1377–79.

12. N. P. Nair et al., "Plasma Melatonin—an Index of Brain Aging in Humans?" *Biological Psychiatry* 21 (1986): 141–50.

13. Ibid.

14. P. E. Kloeden et al., "Artificial Life Extension: The Epigenetic Approach," *Annals of the New York Academy of Science* 719 (May 31, 1994): 474–82.

15. V. M. Dillman et al., "Increase in the Lifespan of Rats Following Polypeptide Pineal Extract Treatment," *Experimental Pathology* 17 (1979): 539–45.

16. Andrew Monjan, personal communication with author, February 1996.

17. Ruth Winter, "The Truth About Antiaging Products," *Consumer's Digest,* 35, no. 3 (May/June 1996): 70.

18. "Melatonin: 'Miracle Hormone' or Media Hype?" *Lifetime Health Letter* (University of Texas, Houston Health Science Center) 7, no. 11 (November 1995): 1.

19. Dillman, "Increase in the Lifespan of Rats."

20. W. B. Mendelson, *Human Sleep: Research and Clinical Care* (New York: Plenum Medical Book Co., 1987), 19.

21. "Getting the Facts About Sleeplessness" (fact sheet from National Sleep Foundation, Washington, D.C., 1996).

22. M. H. Kryger, "Is society sleep deprived" *Sleep* 18, no. 10 (1995): 901; Y. Harrison and J. A. Home, "Should we be taking more sleep?" *Sleep* 18, no. 10 (1995): 901–7; M. H. Sonnet and D. L. Arand, "We are chronically sleep deprived," *Sleep* 18, no. 10 (1995): 908–11.

23. "Sleepless in America: Insomnia Is Widespread," *Lahey Clinic Health Letter,* February 1994, 1–2.

24. Mendleson, *Human Sleep,* 323; "Drugs and Insomnia," NIH Consensus Development Conference report 4, no. 10 (Bethesda, Md., March 26–28, 1990): 2–3; K. Rickels, "The clinical use of hypnotics: indications for use and the need for a variety of hypnotics," *Acta Psychiatry Scandinavia* 74, suppl. 332 (1986): 139.

25. Rickels, "The clinical use of hypnotics," 134.

26. "The Treatment of Sleep Disorders of Older People" (Summary from NIH Consensus Development Conference, National Institutes of Health, Bethesda, Md., March 26–28, 1990).

27. "Sleep Disorders in the Elderly: The Health Consequences" (sponsored by the American Association of Retired Persons and the Upjohn Company, New York, N.Y., October 11, 1988).

28. "Treatment of Sleep Disorders" (NIH Consensus Development Conference).

29. Wilse Webb, *Sleep: The Gentle Tyrant* (Bolton, Mass.: Anker Publishing, 1991), 29–30.

30. William Dement, at News Conference on Insomnia, New York, N.Y., May 15, 1989.

31. Ibid.

32. D. Garfinkel et al., "Improvement of sleep quality in elderly people by controlled-release melatonin," *Lancet* 346 (August 26, 1995): 541–44.

33. Podell, personal communication with author.

34. Bruno Claustrat, "Melatonin and Jet Lag: Confirmatory Result Using a Simplified Protocol," *Biological Psychiatry* 32 (1992): 705–11.

35. Jacqueline Stenson, "Melatonin Not Always What It's Cracked Up to Be," *Medical Tribune News Service,* January 24, 1996.

36. National Institutes of Health Conference on Melatonin, Bethesda, Md., August 12, 1996.

37. Lauren Cerruto, "The Melatonin Controversy," *Neurology Reviews,* November/December 1994, 17.

38. M. W. Miller, "Drug Companies and Health-Food Stores Fight to Peddle Melatonin to Insomniacs," *Wall Street Journal,* August 31, 1994, B1.

39. Ibid.

40. Robert Sack (at Conference on Melatonin at National Institutes of Health, August 12, 1996).

41. Monjan, personal communication with author.

42. E. Friess et al., "DHEA (500 mg) on sleep stages," *American Journal of Physiology* 268, no. 1, pt. 1 (January 1995): E107–13.

43. K. Opstad, "Circadian rhythm of hormones is extinguished during prolonged physical stress, sleep, and energy deficiency in young men," *European Journal of Endocrinology* 131, no. 1 (July 1994): 56–66.

44. E. Friess et al., "The hypothalamic-pituitary-adrenocortical system and sleep in man," *Adv. Neuroimmunology* 5, no. 2 (1995): 111–25.

45. Alexandros Vgontzas, M.D., assistant professor of psychiatry at Penn State's Milton S. Hershey Medical Center, "Chronic Insomnia and Stress Intertwined" (paper presented at the Endocrine Society's 77th annual meeting, Washington, D.C., September 20, 1996).

7: TESTOSTERONE—REPLACEMENT THERAPY AND VIRILITY

1. Robert J. Paradowski, *The American Academic Encyclopedia* (1995 Grolier Multimedia Encyclopedia Version) on CD-ROM, Copyright © 1995 Grolier, Inc., Danbury, Conn.

2. James Hamilton and Gordon Mestler, "Mortality and Survival: A Comparison of Eunuchs with Intact Men and Women" (paper presented at the American Association of Anatomists, Boston, Mass., April 2, 1970).

3. Ibid.

4. *American Encyclopedia* (1995 Grolier Multimedia Version): Peter L. Petrakis; N. R. Moudgal, "Gonadotrophins and Gonadal Function" (1974); B. Runnebaum et al., eds., "Secretion and Action of Gonadotrophins" (1984); B. B. Saxena et al., "Gonadotrophins" (1972).

5. G. Ravaglia, P. Forti, and F. Maioli, "Hormonal Changes in Male Subjects Over Ninety," *Bollettino-Società Italiana Biologia Sperimentale* 71, no. 5–6 (June 1995): 133–39.

6. Ibid.

7. Shalender Bhasin et al., "The Effects of Supraphysiologic Doses of Testosterone on Muscle Size and Strength in Normal Men," *New England Journal of Medicine* 335, no. 1 (July 4, 1996): 1–7.

8. Ibid.

9. Carol K. Yoon, "Scientists Offer Validation Testosterone = Big Muscles," *New York Times,* July 4, 1996, A16.

10. Johns Hopkins release, Baltimore, Md., June 12, 1996.

11. Jean Bolognia, "Aging Skin," *American Journal of Medicine* 98, suppl. 1A (January 16, 1995): 99S–103S.

12. Richard Berger and Deborah Berger, *Biopotency* (Emmaus, Pa.: Rodale Press, 1987).

13. A. Vermeulen and J. M. Kaufman, "Ageing of the Hypothalamo-Pituitary-Testicular Axis in Men," *Hormonal Research* 43, no. 1–3 (1995): 25–28.

14. Ibid.

15. Ibid.

16. Fran Kaiser, "Testosterone Therapy Shows Promise in Elderly Men," *Journal of the American Geriatrics Society,* February 18, 1993.

17. T. J. Aspray et al., "Consequences of withholding testosterone treatment," *Lancet* 348 (August 31, 1996): 609.

18. Fran Kaiser, personal communication with author, February 19, 1996.

19. A. A. Ajayi et al., "Testosterone increases human platelet

thromboxane A2 receptor density and aggregation responses," *Circulation* 91, no. 11 (June 1, 1995): 2742–47.

20. E. L. Barrett-Connor, "Testosterone and risk factors for cardiovascular disease in men," *Diabetes Metabolism* 21, no. 3 (June 1995): 156–61.

21. Kaiser, personal communication with author.

22. *American Encyclopedia* (1995 Grolier Multimedia Version): Julian M. Davidson; R. B. Hochberg and F. Naftolin, "The New Biology of Steroid Hormones" (1991); D. N. Kirk et al., eds., "Dictionary of Steroids" (1991); D. W. Nex and E. J. Parish, eds., "Analysis of Sterols and Other Biologically Significant Steroids" (1989); W. N. Taylor, "Macho Men" (1991).

23. M. A. Kirschner, "Hirsutism and Virilism in Women," *Endocrinology Metabolism* 6 (1984): 55–93.

24. B. Zumoff et al., "Twenty-Four Hour Mean Plasma Testosterone Concentration Declines with Age in Normal Premenopausal Women," *Journal of Endocrinology and Metabolism* 80, no. 4 (April 1995): 1429–30.

25. S. R. Davis et al., "Testosterone enhances estradiol's effects on postmenopausal bone density and sexuality," *Maturitas* 21, no. 3 (April 1995): 227–37.

26. Kaiser, personal communication with author.

27. S. M. Haffner et al., "Decreased testosterone and dehydroepiandrosterone sulfate concentrations are associated with increased insulin and glucose concentrations in nondiabetic men," *Metabolism* 43, no. 5 (May 1994): 599–603.

28. R. Sands and J. Studd, "Exogenous androgens in postmenopausal women," *American Journal of Medicine* 98, no. 1A (January 16, 1995): 76S–79S.

29. Johns Hopkins release, June 12, 1996.

30. Ruth Winter, *A Consumer's Dictionary of Medicines* (New York: Crown Publishers, 1993), 452–53; *Physicians' Desk Reference,* electronic monograph (Montvale, N.J.: Medical Economics Data, 1995).

31. William Masters, "Sex and Aging—Expectations and Reality," *Hospital Practice,* August 15, 1986, 175–92.

8: ESTROGEN—SEXUAL DESIRE, DESIRABILITY, AND ABILITY

1. U.S. Department of Health and Human Services, *Vital Statistics of the United States,* vol. 2, sec. 6, Life Tables (Hyattsville, Md., 1996).

2. J. Kaprio et al., "Common genetic influences on BMI and age at menarche," *Human Biology* 67, no. 5 (October 1995): 739–53; Zaldivar Alvarado et al., "Factors possibly associated with the age at the onset of menopause," *Gynecology and Obstetrics Mexico,* 63 (October 1995): 432–38.

3. Robert A. Wilson and Thelma A. Wilson, "The Fat of the Nontreated Postmenopausal Woman: A Plea for the Maintenance of Adequate Estrogen from Puberty to the Grave," *Journal of the American Geriatrics Society* 11, no. 4 (April 1963): 347–62.

4. K. M. Fox and S. R. Cummings, "Is tubal ligation a risk factor for low bone density and increased risk of fracture?" *American Journal of Obstetrics and Gynecology* 172, no. 1, pt. 1 (January 1995): 101–5.

5. J. A. Cauley et al., "Estrogen Replacement Therapy and Fractures in Older Women," *Annals of Internal Medicine* 122, no. 1 (January 1, 1995): 9–16.

6. Theresa Tamkins, "Taking hormones after menopause may save your teeth," *Medical Tribune News Service,* December 4, 1995.

7. A. Paganini-Hill, "The benefits of estrogen replacement therapy on oral health," *Archives of Internal Medicine* 155, no. 21 (November 27, 1955): 2325–29; M. K. Jeffcoat and C. H. Chestnut 3rd, "Systemic Osteoporosis and Oral Bone Loss: Evidence Shows Increased Risk Factors," *Journal of the American Dentistry Association* 124, no. 11 (November 1993): 49–56.

8. Leon Speroff, "The case for postmenopausal hormone therapy," *Hospital Practice,* February 15, 1996, 75–89; Graham Colditz et al.,

"Menopause and the risk of coronary heart disease in women," *New England Journal of Medicine* 316, no. 18 (April 30, 1987): 1105–9.

9. C. Noel Bairey Merz, speech (at St. Barnabas Medical Center's Medical Education Department meeting cosponsored by Wyeth-Ayerst, West Orange, N.J., June 5, 1996).

10. "Mixture May Rival Estrogen in Preventing Heart Disease," Associated Press, August 15, 1996.

11. Margo Denke, "Combined Hormone Therapy Lowers Cholesterol and Uterine-Cancer Risk," *Southwestern Medical Center at Dallas News Report,* August 22, 1996.

12. S. M. Haffner et al., "Relation of Sex Hormones and Dehydro-epiandrosterone Sulfate (DHEA-SO4) to cardiovascular risk factors in postmenopausal women," *American Journal of Epidemiology* 142, no. 9 (November 1, 1995): 925–34.

13. University of Medicine and Dentistry of New Jersey press release, May 23, 1989.

14. Raul Raz and Walter Stamm, "A Controlled Trial of Intravaginal Estriol in Postmenopausal Women With Recurrent Urinary Tract Infections," *New England Journal of Medicine* 329 (1993): 753–56.

15. Masters, "Sex and Aging."

16. Abrams, Berkow, and Fletcher, *Merck Manual of Geriatrics,* 586.

17. Ibid., 586, 837.

18. Ibid., 838.

19. Karen Steinberg, Stephen Thacker et al., "A Meta-analysis of the Effect of Estrogen Replacement Therapy on the Risk of Breast Cancer," *Journal of the American Medical Association* 1991, no. 265 (1985–1990): 361–71.

20. H. Fillit, "Future Therapeutic Developments of Estrogen Use," *Journal of Clinical Pharmacology* (September 1995) and 35(9Suppl): 25S–28S, speech before St. Barnabas Medical Center's Medical Education Department meeting, cosponsored by Wyeth-Ayerst, June 5, 1996, West Orange, New Jersey.

21. Francine Grodstein et al., "Prospective Study of Exogenous

Hormones and Risk of Pulmonary Embolism in Women," *Lancet* 348 (October 12, 1996): 983–87.

22. Louis Kuritzky, *Hospital Practice,* May 15, 1995, 24k–24q.

23. Eugenia E. Calle, H. L. Miracle-McMahill, M. J. Thun and C. W. Health, "Estrogen Replacement Therapy and Risk of Fatal Colon Cancer," *Journal of The National Cancer Institute,* 87, no. 7 (April 5, 1995): 517–23.

24. "Estrogen Replacement Therapy May Increase Women's Risk of Fatal Ovarian Cancer," American Cancer Society News Service release, May 1, 1995.

25. G. A. Colditz et al., "The Use of Estrogen and Progestins and the Risk of Breast Cancer in Postmenopausal Women," *New England Journal of Medicine* 332 (1995): 1589–93.

26. J. L. Stanford et al., "Combined estrogen and progestin hormone replacement therapy in relation to risk of breast cancer in middle-aged women," *Journal of the American Medical Association* 274, no. 2 (July 12, 1995): 178–79.

27. Collaborative Group on Hormonal Factors in Breast Cancer, "Breast cancer and hormonal contraceptives: collaborative reanalysis of individual data on 53,297 women with breast cancer and 100,239 women without breast cancer from 54 epidemiological studies," *Lancet* 347 (1996): 1713–27.

28. Karen Steinberg et al., "A Meta-Analysis of the Effect of Estrogen Replacement Therapy on the Risk of Breast Cancer," *Journal of the American Medical Association* 265, no. 15 (April 17, 1991): 1985–90.

29. Colditz et al., "The Use of Estrogen and Progestins."

30. *American Medical Association News,* May 13, 1996, 18.

31. Gerson Weiss, speech (at St. Barnabas Medical Center's Medical Education Department and Wyeth-Ayerst cosponsored meeting, West Orange, N.J., June 5, 1996).

32. Stephen Barnes, "The Isoflavone Genistein: A Good Reason for Eating Soy" (paper presented at the 208th American Cancer Society National Meeting, Washington, D.C.. August 21, 1994).

33. National Institutes of Health, National Institute on Aging, *Menopause* (Washington, D.C.: NIH Publication No. 94-3886, 1995).

34. Claudia Wallis, "The Estrogen Dilemma," *Time,* June 26, 1995, 46–52.

35. Ibid.

36. Annlia Paganini-Hill, personal communication with author, August 20, 1996.

37. *UCLA Berkeley Wellness Letter,* October 1995, 4.

38. Barbara Wich and Molly Carnes, "Menopause and the Aging Female Reproductive System," *Endocrinology and Metabolism Clinics of America* 24, no. 2 (June 1995): 273–95.

ⁿ P.A. Newcomb and B.E. Storer, "Postmenopausal hormone use and risk of large-bowel cancer," *Journal of the National Cancer Institute,* 1995 Jul 19, 1987(14):1039–40.

9: Aiding Brain Function and Brightening Mood

1. *Lancet,* August 17, 1996.

2. "Estrogen May Reduce Alzheimer's Risk in Women, Study Says," *New York Times,* August 16, 1996, A18.

3. Joan Stephenson, "More Evidence Links NSAID, Estrogen Use With Reduced Alzheimer's Risk," *Journal of the American Medical Association* 275, no. 18 (May 8, 1996): 1389–90.

4. Ohkura, "Evaluation of estrogen treatment in Female Patients with Dementia of Alzheimer's type," *Journal of Endocrinology* 41, no. 4 (August 1994): 361–71.

5. V. W. Henderson et al., "Estrogen replacement therapy in older women. Comparison between Alzheimer's disease cases and nondemented control subjects," *Archives of Neurology* 51, no. 9 (1994): 896–900.

6. Paganini-Hill, personal communication with author.

7. McNeil, "Alzheimer's Disease,"

8. Frank Bellino, personal communication with author, August 19, 1996.

9. H. Fillit, "Future Therapeutic Developments of Estrogen Use,"

Journal of Clinical Pharmacology (September 1995) and 35 (9 Suppl): 255–285, speech before St. Barnabas Medical Center's Medical Education Department meeting, June 5, 1996.

10. Stephenson, "More Evidence Links NSAID, Estrogen Use."

11. Michael Gooch and Douglass Stennett, "Molecular Basis of Alzheimer's Disease," *American Journal of Health-System Pharmacists* 53 (July 1, 1996), 1545–47.

12. Ibid.

13. Douglass Stennett, personal communication with author, August 15, 1996.

14. Stephenson, "More Evidence Links NSAID, Estrogen Use."

15. Johns Hopkins release, Baltimore, Md., June 14, 1996.

16. Marianne Hassler, "Testosterone and Artistic Talents," *International Journal of Neuroscience* 56 (1991): 25–38.

17. Sandra Blakeslee, "Female Sex Hormone Is Tied to Ability to Perform Tasks," *New York Times,* November 18, 1988, 1.

18. Marc Blackman, personal communication with author, August 20, 1996.

19. Merill, Harrington, and Sunderland, "Reduced Plasma Dehydroepiandrosterone Concentration," 102–5.

20. Eugene Roberts and L. Jaime Fitten, "Serum Steroid Levels in Two Old Men with Alzheimer's Disease," in *Biologic Role of Dehydroepiandrosterone,* 43–61.

21. Kenneth Bonnet and Richard Brown, "Cognitive Effects of DHEA Replacement Therapy," in *Biologic Role of Dehydroepiandrosterone,* 65–78.

22. Y. Sheline et al., "Hippocampal atrophy in Recurrent Major Depression," *Proceedings of the National Academy of Sciences USA* 93, no. 3908 (1996).

23. J. D. Bremner et al., "MRI-based measurement of hippocampal volume in patients with Post-traumatic Stress Disorder," *American Journal of Psychiatry* 152 (1995): 973–81.

24. Arthur Winter and Ruth Winter, *Build Your Brain Power* (New York: St. Martin's Press, 1986) 160–64.

25. J. W. Newcomer, S. Craft et al., "Glucocorticoid-Induced Impairment in Declarative Memory Performance in Adult Humans," *Journal of Neuroscience* 14, no. 4 (April 1994): 2047–53.

26. National Institutes of Health, *Menopause*.

27. Ibid.

28. L. Uzych, "Anabolic-androgenic steroids and psychiatric-related effects: A review," *Canadian Journal of Psychiatry* 37, no. 1 (February 1992): 23–28.

29. Villareal and Morley, "Trophic Factors in Aging."

30. B. B. Sherwin, "Sex hormones and psychological functioning in postmenopausal women," *Experimental Gerontology* 29, no. 304 (May-August 1994): 423–30.

31. Regelson, Kalimi, and Loria, "DHEA: Some Thoughts."

32. J. F. Flood, et al., "Memory enhancing effects in male mice of pregnenolone and steroids metabolically derived from it," *Proceedings of the National Academy of Sciences* 89 (March 1992): 1567–71; H. Freeman et al., "Therapeutic efficacy of delta-5 pregnenolone in rheumatoid arthritis," *Journal of the American Medical Association,* April 15, 1950; 1124–28; M. Warner and J. A. Gustafsson, "Cytochromone P450 in the brain: neuroendocrine functions," *Frontiers of Neuroendocrinology* 16, no. 3 (July 1995): 224–36.

33. L. Guth et al., "Key role for pregnenolone in combination therapy that promotes recovery after spinal cord injury," *Neurobiology* 91 (December 1994): 12308–12.

34. J. F. Flood et al., "Age-related decrease of plasma testosterone in SAMP8 mice: replacement improves age-related impairment of learning and memory," *Physiology of Behavior* 57, no. 4 (April 1995): 669–73; Fran Kaiser, personal communication with author, August 22, 1996.

35. J. F. Flood et al., "Memory enhancing effects in male mice of pregnenolone and steroids metabolically derived from it," *Proceedings of The National Academy of Sciences* 89 (March 1992) 1567–71; H. Freeman et al., "Therapeutic efficacy of delta-5 pregnenolone in rheumatoid arthritis," *Journal of The American Medical*

Association, April 15, 1950, 1124–28; M. Warner, J. A. Gustafsson, "Cytochromone P450 in the brain: neuroendocrine functions," *Frontiers of Neuroendocrinology 1995* 16, no. 3 (July 1995): 224–36.

36. L. Guth et al., "Key Role for pregnenolone in combination therapy that promotes recovery after spinal cord injury." *Neurobiology* 91 (December 1994): 12308–12.

37. R. H. Purdy et al., "Stress-induced elevations of gamma-aminobutyric acid Type A receptor-active steroids in the rat brain" *Proceedings of the National Academy of Sciences* 88 (December 29, 1995): 4553–57; F. Holsboer et al., "Steroid effects on central neurons and implications for psychiatric and neurological disorders," *Annals of the New York Academy of Sciences* 746 (November 30, 1994): 345–59.

38. J. F. Flood, S. A. Farr, F. E. Kaiser, M. La Regina, and J. E. Morley, "Age-related decrease of plasma testosterone in SAMP8 mice: replacement improves age-related impairment of learning and memory," *Physiology of Behavior 1995,* 57, no. 4 (April): 669–73; Fran Kaiser, MD, personal communication with author, August 22, 1996.

39. Harris Lieberman et al., "Effects of Melatonin on Human Mood and Performance," *Brain Research* 323 (1984): 201–7.

40. G. M. Brown, "Psychoneuroendocrinology," *Psychiatric Journal of the University of Ottawa* 14, no. 2 (1989): 344–48.

41. Ibid.

42. Ibid.

43. Joel Davis, *Endorphins* (New York: Dial Press, 1984).

44. Alma Guinness, ed., *ABC's of the Human Mind* (Pleasantville, N.Y.: Reader's Digest Association Books, 1990), 28.

10: ANTI-AGING HORMONE RESEARCH AND YOUR MORE YOUTHFUL FUTURE

1. V. A. Lesnikov, W. Pierpaoli, "Pineal cross-transplantation (old-to-young and vice versa) as evidence for an endogenous aging clock,"

Annals of The New York Academy of Sciences 719 (May 31, 1994): 456–60.

2. Michael S. Jazwinskin, "Longevity, Genes, and Aging," *Science* 273 (July 5, 1996): 54–63.

3. Phyllis Wise et al., "Menopause: The Aging of Multiple Pacemakers," *Science* 273 (July 5, 1996): 67–70.

INDEX

Acetylcholine, 70, 195, 213, 214

Adams, Gregg A., 79

Addison, Thomas, 16

Addison's disease, 16, 17

Adipostat, 93–95

Adrenal glands, 3, 203
  adrenopause, 16–17
  cortex, 14, 16
  functions of, 6
  medulla, 14
  overproduction of, 204
  stress and, 13–15
  see also specific glands

Adrenergic hormones, 213

Adrenocorticotropic hormone
  (ACTH), 9, 14, 203

Advanced Tissue Sciences, 66

AIDS, 41
  DHEA and, 25
  growth factors and, 75, 76–77
  Serostim and, 61
  testosterone and, 146–47

Allele-type 4, 197, 198

Allergic reactions, 40

Alzheimer's disease, 192–205,
  214
  DHEA and, 202–205
  estrogen and, 192–99
  NGF and, 70–72, 195
  testosterone and, 199–202

*American Dental Association
  Journal,* 167

American Journal of Medicine,
  148, 154

Amygdala, 207

Amyotrophic lateral sclerosis
  (ALS), 68–69

Anabolic steroids, 138, 144–47
  AIDS and, 146–47
  athletes and, 144–45, 146
  as a controlled drug, 145
  increasing strength and, 145–46
  mood and, 210
  to promote recovery, 144
  side effects of, 144, 146
  synthetic, 143
  see also Testosterone

Andrews, William, 89–90, 186